U0338478

为什么？

在父母选择自杀后的日子里
WHEN BOTH MY PARENTS TOOK THEIR LIVES

（新加坡）尹 著　　钟耀林 译

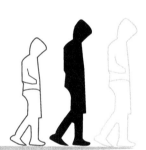

中国经济出版社
CHINA ECONOMIC PUBLISHING HOUSE
北 京

图书在版编目（CIP）数据

为什么？：在父母选择自杀后的日子里：汉、英／（新加坡）尹著；
钟耀林译．—北京：中国经济出版社，2017.7
ISBN 978 - 7 - 5136 - 4632 - 1

Ⅰ.①为… Ⅱ.①尹… ②钟… Ⅲ.①精神疗法—通俗读物—汉、英
Ⅳ.①R749.055 - 49

中国版本图书馆 CIP 数据核字（2017）第 050247 号

Originally published in English in 2008 by Epigram Books.
1008 Toa Payoh North #03 - 08 Singapore 318996
Tel：+65 6292 4456/Fax：+65 6292 4414
enquiry@ epigrambooks. sg/www. epigrambooks. sg
著作权合同登记号：图字01 - 2017 - 3941 号

责任编辑　叶亲忠
责任印制　马小宾
封面设计　华子设计

出版发行　中国经济出版社
印 刷 者　北京九州迅驰传媒文化有限公司
经 销 者　各地新华书店
开　　本　710mm×1000mm　1/16
印　　张　11.5
字　　数　170 千字
版　　次　2017 年 7 月第 1 版
印　　次　2019 年 4 月第 2 次
定　　价　38.00 元

广告经营许可证　京西工商广字第 8179 号

中国经济出版社 网址 www. economyph. com 社址 北京市西城区百万庄北街 3 号 邮编 100037
本版图书如存在印装质量问题，请与本社发行中心联系调换（联系电话：010 - 68330607）

此书献给我的父亲和母亲，以此怀念他们。即使他们现在已永远地离开了我，但他们将永恒地活在我的心里、我的记忆里。

　　另外，我要将此书献给新加坡援人协会的首席执行官——玛丽·马修女士。她的温暖和善解人意给了我面对双亲自杀身亡考验的希望。

前　言

当我们所爱的人死于自杀，留给我们的将是如何挽救破碎的心这一痛苦的考验。这让我们精神上饱受创伤，还有留给关于如何合理化解释自杀以及重新生活的巨大挑战。

在自杀事件发生后，遗属们失去亲人和遭受巨大悲痛，还往往被误解，有时候，身边的人也会提供一些不恰当的安慰和支持。他们想帮忙，但是往往帮倒忙，反而像在伤口上撒盐，增加了遗属的痛苦和悲伤。

对遗属来说，自杀事件发生后，要他们去接受、欣赏和适应生活同样是个巨大的挑战。很多人选择沉默不语和孤独去面对所发生的事情，结果走不出来。

或许我们要做的是让这些遗属们发声，倾听他们艰辛的疗愈故事。这也是尹的意图——和我们一起分享她以及和她一样的遗属们的故事。

我认为，能够和尹一起经历这段疗愈之旅，是新加坡援人协会的荣幸。最吸引人的地方是她真诚的坦露，吸引我们进入她的内心世界，体验她在父亲自杀后作为遗属是如何疗愈内心创伤的。

这份来自尹的第一手叙事记录，不仅旨在启发读者，同时也作为镇痛药，给正遭受丧亲之痛的同伴以支持。

　　我很感激尹为新加坡援人协会所做的贡献，同时也感激其他所有对遗属伸出疗愈之手的同伴们。

　　希望你也能和尹以及她的同伴们一样，与那些正经历迷失和悲痛的遗属一起分享这本书。

新加坡援人协会主席及顾问

安东尼·杨

咨询与护理中心治疗师

序　言

父亲自杀让我淹没于伤心、悲痛和遗憾之中。我的情绪犹如过山车般变化起伏，我感到极度迷失。一位朋友建议我到新加坡援人协会去接受咨询辅导。克服了内心无数次的抵抗和犹豫，我拨通了援人协会的热线，随后便发现自己很快就进入了一段痛苦、疲倦却是不可或缺的疗愈旅程。

提出写这本书的是我的咨询师奥菲利娅。最初我是不情愿的，这和写日记不一样，写日记我可随心所欲地表达，尽情地把压抑我的事情写下来。应付那些翻滚的回忆对我来说本来就已经够难的了。撰写一本关于父亲自杀的书意味着要回忆过去痛苦的记忆，就像重新经历一场噩梦。坐下来，回忆并记录过去所发生的一切，这样的事情想想都觉得恐怖。写这本书的畏惧表现在我的拖延之中。我告诉自己要写关于父亲自杀的书太痛苦了，我又不是作家，我的野心是不是太大了，居然还想写本书。我从未做过这么大的工程。但另一个我告诉自己，这或许是我从苦海中提炼一点点有用的东西的一条路，这或许能给那些遭受家人自杀创伤、倍感孤独的遗属们一些慰藉。

最初，我甚至连"自杀"这个词都写不出来。每当我使用这个词的时候，父亲自杀的事实就闯进我的内心，占据我的头脑。悲伤吞没了我，在写作上我集中不了一丝精力。我重新使用字母"s"代替，直至我有足够勇气在电脑屏幕中看到这个词语。

我曾经一度想要完全中断这个计划，因为在撰写过程中，我被带到了悲伤的深处。但是，回眸过去，我庆幸自己能坚持写完这本书。因为在撰写过程中，写作变得越来越具有疗愈力。写作给予了我情感和思维上全新的出口。当我想要记录所发生的一切和心中所想，我会把时间花在撰写上。当我想要休息片刻，我会选择停下来。当然，在这过程中满是泪水。但其中也有许多令我开心的回忆，我回想起父亲的慈祥和温和，还有父女间美好的经历，这些时刻都让我感到父亲的万千宠爱和幸福。

撰写这本书也是一段生命之旅，在这过程中我发现了自己生命中不曾被看到过的部分。我必须说明我并非在炫耀自己的这些发现，但现在的我更了解自己，也学会了多爱护自己一些。

因此，我要把这本书作为礼物，献给我自己及所有遗属。

作者　尹

译 者 序

第一次看到这本书是在 2015 年 4 月，那时我正参加新加坡社会工作服务考察。当时新加坡援人协会（SOS）的工作人员郑重地向我们推介了这本书。我翻书浏览，很快就被书中作者的故事打动了。与其说这是一段苦难史，还不如说它是一部坚强史。这更是一本难得的疗愈之书，来自作者作为案主的第一手叙事，这一点让它显得更加珍贵。这样的书籍，至少目前在中国国内还很少见到。于是，我当场便坐不住了，也不顾自己蹩脚的英文水平，厚颜请缨，想把这本书翻译到国内，介绍给国内的读者。

本书的原作者尹在 7 岁的时候，母亲死于自杀。40 年后，她父亲从公寓的楼上跳了下去。内心巨大的悲伤、耻辱、怨恨和愤怒，还有各种来自亲友、旁人的不理解、指责，让尹喘不过气来。幸运的是，在尹的生命历程中有丈夫、孩子、友人以及新加坡援人协会的工作人员和同为遗属的一帮"疗愈桥"小组组员的支持和陪伴，让尹一步一步地从生命的低谷中走了出来。

细读本书，您将会被带入尹的生命故事当中，为她的失去扼腕痛惜，为她的痛苦热泪盈眶，为她的抗争感动，也为她的突破而欣喜。同时我还要告诉您，这不仅仅是一本记叙尹经历的故事书，这更是一部记载作者在穿越苦难中呐喊、对生命意义深层体验的疗愈之书。所以我希望把这本书推送给所有的社工同行和心理学爱好者，尤其希望推荐给正处于家人自杀或重大家庭变故阴霾中的遗属们。

如果您是助人工作的同行，本书最大的作用莫过于案主在书中清晰细腻地描述了自己从遭受创伤到实现疗愈的过程，从抗拒、畏缩到试一下、不配合和一步步走向康复。这些难得的第一手叙事资料真实、细腻，有助于我们更好地了解案主的内心世界，思考如何能够从案主自身出发，挖掘案主内在的生命动力，以实现疗愈。

如果您是正处于家人自杀或重大家庭变故阴霾中的遗属，面对亲人离去，或是悲痛，或是愤怒，或是自责，或是怨恨，或是兼而有之。如何找到一条路，走出这困境？本书将给大家介绍一个个鲜活的例子。作者的经历和心路历程可能会是我们的一个模板。当悲剧发生，很多人选择了沉默，希望以此忘记所有不开心的事情。可是深深地烙在心头的这份悲痛无法被岁月带走。那我们能怎么办？记得台湾叙事疗愈王子周志建先生曾这样比喻，我们要做的不是要忘记那个不开心的自己，而是要学会安顿内心那个受伤的小孩，学会与他和平相处。学会安顿内心那个受伤的小孩，学会拥抱生活，接纳自己，接纳已经发生的事情，勇敢地面对人生，这或许才是处理生命伤痛故事的一种比较现实的方法。

本书的翻译出版，并非一帆风顺。首先翻译过程断断续续，那是因为作者的生命故事不断地激起了我内心的波澜。作者所经受的，和我这几年因为父亲癌病离开人世所遇到的困惑有几分相似。在用有限的英文水平翻译的过程中，我不断尝试走进作者的内心世界，但每每如此，涌起的对作者的痛惜、同情和欣喜，也间接折射到了自己的人生经历中。这几年，因为对苦难的困惑，我开始对叙事产生了兴趣，并撰写了《癌病与持续性的痛——我的叙事疗愈行动》一书。在新加坡考察时，接触到新加坡援人协会，当他们推荐尹的这本书时，我当下就决定一定要把这本书翻译到国内，希望推送给国内的朋友。可以说《为什么？——在父母选择自杀后的日子里》这本书和《癌病与持续性的痛——我的叙事疗愈行动》是我叙事疗愈路上的姊妹篇。

版权联系也几经波折，在这里要诚挚地感谢新加坡援人协会（SOS）在此书的翻译出版过程中真诚无私的帮助；感谢 EPIGRAM 出版社 Req Ang 和他的一帮同事，前后与我互通近百封邮件，不厌其烦地协助处理版权事宜；说到这里，还要特别感谢为本书翻译出版费尽心思的中国经济出版社叶亲忠先生和他的一帮同事，几经周折，最终完成所有的手续。

说到致谢，当然少不了要感谢原作者，是她向我们敞开心扉，给我们指出一条通往疗愈的路；还要感谢广东省社会工作教育与实务协会，不辞辛苦地链接新加坡社会服务资源；还要感谢在翻译前期做了大量工作的岭南师范学院的同学，他们是陈凯铃、麦敏君、谢瑞妃、刘沛文、黄家欣、魏恬祯、刘娇芬等；另外，还有很多同仁为本书的翻译出版提过诸多宝贵意见，来不及一一致谢，在此一并谢过！

由于翻译能力有限，加上中国和新加坡两地文化的差异，书中不免有所纰漏，敬请各位读者海涵赐教！经叶亲忠先生提议，两地出版社协商，中英文合并出版，以慰读者！

此谢！

钟耀林

2017 年 2 月

目　录

第一章

父亲，为什么？

我们在位于广东民弄的新加坡援助协会（SOS）办公室的一个房间里见面。一双双好奇的眼睛透过窗帘往室外偷偷窥探着，似乎在寻找着什么。在我们前方的桌子上摆着一些饮品和纸巾。我们去那是为了分享我们那段痛苦不堪的故事。我期待自己的出现能给其他同样曾经遭受不幸经历的人带来一些安慰。当他们讲述自己的痛苦、无助、空虚和起伏不定的情绪时，我能够理解他们，因为曾经我和他们一样，也有过如此痛苦绝望的经历。我在认真聆听他们故事的过程中，清楚地意识到，给予这些遗属支持，是在这场孤独且令人畏惧的旅程中最重要的。但与此同时，出现在那里，我被卷回到成为遗属的宿命般的那天——父亲自杀那天。那一天是我终点不明、孤独旅程的开始。

在那天以前

在父亲自杀以前将近两年的时间里，他的状况一直都不是很好。他已接近 90 岁高龄了，在每周的探访中，我都注意到他整体的健康状况在逐渐地衰退——他的身体持续出现痛苦和不适，想必这也是导致了他选择自杀的关键原因。他身体很虚弱，情感和心灵也很脆弱，同时饱受精神上的挑战。对父亲而言，他的祈祷并没有得到上帝的回应，他对于自己的身体状态也逐渐变得气馁和沮丧。此时的他对未来充满了恐惧。

老年医学专家对父亲做出的诊断是伴随早期痴呆倾向的抑郁症。频繁地看医生并没有太多地减轻他对疾病的抱怨。看着父亲的病情逐渐恶化，身体大不如前，我伤心得难以言表。很多时候，当我们聊天时，他屡次向我诉说，渴望上帝能带走他，带他飞往天堂。他已经厌倦了这样的生活。

我心底里知道他是在想我的母亲了，非常想念。他鳏居多年，长期孤独。他时常思念母亲。他们是包办婚姻，当初在还没见到母亲本人以前，父亲就同意娶她了。母亲是父亲心中那个陪伴他多年、漂亮的并且在中国完成高中学业的贤妻。母亲逝世以后被火葬，她的骨灰被安置在骨灰库里，父亲预定了一个紧挨母亲骨灰旁的壁龛，希望将来用来存放他的骨灰，想到等上帝带走他时，和母亲葬在一起。但是，上帝并没有如他所愿，也没有听到我的祈祷，没有让父亲永生没有痛苦。我曾认为让上帝听见我们的祷告只是时间问题。但让我万万没想到的是，父亲已经秘密地决定要离开这个世界到另外一个世界去，以至于他能和上帝、和母亲在一起了。

父亲和我的关系十分密切，我也从来没有想象过失去他的生活会是怎样的，即使在我的潜意识里，我早已意识到他年事已高，健康状况欠佳。7岁那年，我失去了母亲，他身兼父职和母职照顾我，为我做饭，送我上学。即使在我叛逆的青春期里，他的父爱也不曾动摇过。在我的童年里，他是我的知己；而在他垂暮之年，我俩变换了角色——我又成了他的知己。他的离世不是因为疾病或高龄，而是因为他选择了以自杀的方式来结束自己的生命，这让我很崩溃。

那一天

宿命般的那一天像平常的周末一样照常运转。送完孩子上学后，我照旧去了水产市场，买了条新鲜的鱼，带回给父亲的保姆，让她做给父亲吃。当我到达父亲公寓的时候，父亲仍然躺在床上——虽然那段时间他几乎无时无刻都躺在床上，但却昼夜失眠。我们聊了一会，我尝试着振作他的精神。但在内心深处，我像往常一样感到无助，因为我知道他正经历着非常困难的时期，我做不了任何事情来安慰他。父亲很重视个人的独立，所以他不愿意接受别人的帮助。但现在他已经到了非常时期，必须要依靠他人的帮助来完成日常行动，甚至是最基本的个人小事。这让他的自尊很受伤。他开始变得抑郁了。

由于失眠，父亲缺乏足够的休息，他开始变得偏执，对周围的人都不信任，做什么事情都不高兴。我意识到，生活对他来说已经毫无意义了，他越来越无法忍受继续活下去的生活。这段时期由于要适应他的这种行为变化，我过得很困难。父亲过去是一个很理性、富有激情、友好、温和、信奉上帝、有信仰以及有很多性格优点的人。我为父亲在他生命的这个时候失去这些感到伤心。即使他依旧活着，但他已经不再是我认识的那个父亲了。但我知道在这个时候，他最需要我的关心和理解。于是，我暗自决定，尽自己最大的努力让他在剩余的日子里尽可能过得好受和舒适一点。

那一天，像往常那样，我坐在父亲的床上和他谈话，给他念每天的新闻，尝试让他提起点兴趣，然后哄他入睡，我们的角色互换了——我像一个母亲那样对他，而他就像小孩。我多么希望时光能回到从前，回到他年轻力壮的时候。

不管我做了多少努力去安慰他、哄他睡觉，但他还是难以入眠。他告诉我，他没胃口，总感到疲倦。我给他喂了点浓缩鸡汤，希望这能使他强壮起来，哪怕就只是今天。由于我不得不去做其他事情，我告诉他我必须要走了，改天再来看他。当他和我说"再见"的时候，他看起来和往常没什么不同。然而，那却是我最后一次亲手喂父亲吃饭，最后一次和他亲密接触，最后一次能听到他的声音，最后一次看到他活着的模样。那个场景，那段最后一次接触的记忆，我永远也不会忘记——我们各自道了最后的一声"再见"。

几个小时后，当我在做其他事情的时候，我接到大哥的来电。他和父亲住在一起，因此他来电一般都是和我聊聊父亲和他的最新状况。有时，他只是发泄作为一名主要照顾者的沮丧和无助。所以，我继续开着车，准备戴上耳塞听他讲话。

"父亲跳下去了"，他说。我简直无法相信我所听到的。

"他已经跳下去了，你说的是什么意思？"这个消息重重地打击了我，我停下车，并把车往公路边上靠。我的心跳得很快，我陷入了极度的恐惧当中。我记得，电话那头传来了尖叫声和哭泣声，还有一连串质问哥哥的问题："为什么会这样？怎么会发生这种事情的？保姆在哪里？为什么她没有阻止他？"

闪现在我脑海中的场景是父亲跳下去之前的最后片刻。他是怎样挪到窗户边的？早上我离开的时候他身体是如此的虚弱，几乎连坐在床上的力气也没有，他是怎么爬上窗台的？他一定是使尽了全身的力量，想方设法去完成最后一项体力活。我脑海里反复涌现他跳下去的场景，我无法摆脱那恐怖的画面。一连串的问题在我脑海里涌现出来。为什么会发生这种事？为什么他想自杀？为什么我没有预见？为什么他要放弃？为什么他不告诉我？为什么他要以这种方式离开？天啊！他一定是遭受了极大的痛苦。我肯定的是，如果他没有饱受极度的绝望和折磨，他是不会选择这种悲剧的方式（来结束自己生命的①）。想到父亲生前饱受精神上的折磨，我感到无法言表的痛苦。

在车上，我拨通了丈夫办公室的电话。他急忙赶过来，我们一起开车前往父亲的公寓。一路上，强烈的愧疚感、后悔和一种彻底的失落感波涛般地向我涌来，给我当头一棒。与此同时，我根本无法相信父亲自杀已成事实。

当我们到达父亲公寓的时候，我无法让自己去看他的身体。这种事情怎么会发生呢？早上明明他还活着，怎么现在就永远地离开这个世界了呢？然而事实是冷酷的、残忍的，简单明了得超乎了我身、心、灵上的理解能力。此时的我好像被撕裂成了两半，一个我想要见到他、去触摸他、和他在一起，另一个我却想逃离这儿。我不想去证实这些，我不忍面对父亲的遗体，不忍面对他已逝的事实，我极度希望能继续相信父亲他还活着。我非常害怕我所看到的，我还能认出他来吗？他的遗体会是残缺不全和血肉模糊的吗？我会不会到处见到他的身体器官呢？

在知道父亲死讯后，我联系了和我关系亲密的朋友蒂娜，她赶了过来。在混乱和害怕中，我问蒂娜我是否应该去看我父亲的遗体。她不同意，她害怕我无法面对我所看到的事实。她让我仔细冷静地考虑，对我而言，记住父亲早期活着的模样是否比记住他躺在草地上的样子会更好一些。现今，我很庆幸当初听从了她的意见，因为在我脑海里，还保留着父亲活着时的模样，健康而完整。

警察在事发现场开展调查。在父亲的公寓里，他们聚集在父亲跳下去

---

① 译者注

的那扇窗户的周围。紧挨着窗户的是一张凳子，凳子旁是我父亲的拖鞋，窗户的边缘遗留了父亲的另一只拖鞋，那是父亲跳下去的时候落下的。隔着一段距离，我看到警察他们好像在商议什么。我就好像在看一场电影，而我自己并没有真正的在里面。我只是躯体在那里，但我又觉得我离得很远。在一定程度上，只有在有人和我说话的时候，我才意识我也在其中。即使是这样，我也感觉好像另一个自己在答话。

警察当然有他们的工作要做，然而，无论如何他们的出现对一个正处于悲伤之中的家庭来说都是一种打扰。他们以一种冷漠而专业的方式问各种问题，而他们所问的大部分都指向保姆，因为她是最后见到父亲还活着的人。在调查结束后，他们对父亲的遗体要在第二天送到太平间的要求作了一些程序上的指导，然后就离开了。

每一起自杀事件警察都要介入。为了排除他杀的可能，通常来说验尸必须要做。他脆弱的身体被解剖开的想法是多么的难以想象。即使曾经听说过验尸如何开展的恐怖故事，似乎也毫无帮助，因为这些想法早已袭击着我那早已脆弱不堪的情绪。父亲生前总是那么整洁和得体，但是现在有一群陌生人看着他赤裸的躯体并且要解剖他。他们能以他应得的尊重来对待他的身体吗？对父亲的尸检，我感到极度的无助。我束手无策，没有办法保护他，无法控制这种事情的发生。这样的想法看似缺乏理性，但我在想父亲在那里该多冷啊，没有人给他温暖。当父亲还活着的时候，他不喜欢到冰冷的地方，然而太平间却是一个非常冷的地方。

我的哥哥们给了我一项任务，让我为父亲挑选寿衣。我是父亲三个孩子中最年幼的一个，也是唯一的女儿，跟父亲最亲近。这件事让我感到极其伤心和为难。这真的很离奇，今早父亲还活得好好的，而现在，我却要为他挑选最后穿着进棺材的衣服。为什么事情会变成这样？所发生的这一切是多么不可理喻。

我要怎么应对这样的痛苦？我怎么样才能在父亲死于自杀这一永远挥之不去的巨大阴影之中活下来呢？我怎么样才能面对我将不再感到快乐的生活？毫无意义的生存将会是怎样的？我怎么样才能生活在父亲被痛苦折磨以至于自杀的思绪中？以一种极端的方式逃离这种痛苦的念头一闪而过，那就是选择和父亲一样的路——尝试去自杀，这样就能逃离我将要面对的痛苦了。

那晚回家后，我感到精疲力竭，觉得整个人的情绪、心灵、精神都被摧残了，我尝试去休息，却徘徊在半睡半醒之间。

第二天

当我醒来的第二天，整个人都感到麻木和毫无知觉。记忆中，我若无其事般地去找理发师梳洗头发。我和理发师的谈话和从前毫无差别，一切照常。理发师也没有觉察到我有任何的悲伤和疲倦。如从前般，她问起我父亲的健康状况，我也像往常一样回答：父亲渐渐变老了，身体很虚弱。

理完发后，我还去了杂货店购物。我在过道上来回走着，挑选了一些日常的家庭用品，购物出奇地分散了我的注意力。我做着往常的事情，似乎所有的事情一切都很顺利。我还给我的一个朋友打了电话，让她替我保守父亲离世的秘密，不要让我圈子里其他的朋友知道，因为我想为父亲办一个清静的葬礼。在通话过程中，我很冷静，很镇定，就像是从别人口中说出他们需要告知别人的事情一样，而不是我本人在说话。我感觉自己并不在现场一样。

一整天我的两个哥哥给我打了许多通电话，问我关于父亲的丧礼安排和讣闻位置的意见。难以解释的是我能够以一种超然的镇定接听每通电话。我知道"麻木"也是自我保护的本能反应。我在现实世界和超现实的世界间游移不定，同时夹杂了其他的紧张激烈的情绪。当我在现实和超现实的世界中摇摆不定，尝试着弄清楚那些正在发生的事情时，我感到精疲力竭。我知道父亲是死于自杀，但是，在那时，父亲自杀的全部影响并没有从情感上彻底击垮我。当我能着手做必须要完成的事情时，在我潜意识的某个地方，我知道有悲剧已经发生了，但要我逐渐适应这件事情却是何等的困难。因此，当我独自一人待着的时候，或者和不知道父亲已离世的朋友待在一起的时候，我表现得很正常。

然而，现实终究是现实，不久之后的那个下午，我被告知要去接收父亲的棺材。那一刻，我再也无法否认父亲永远地离开了我这个事实。父亲死了，躺在棺材里一动不动，这样的场景彻底粉碎了我对另一个世界的臆想，在那个世界里，父亲老了，身体还是很虚弱，但仍然活着。我一直在死守着一个期望，希望这所有的一切都只是一场噩梦，而当我醒来的时候，一切照常。但令我极度悲伤的是，这不是一场噩梦，再也不存在什么希望。

全家人按照指示站到守灵的地方。这将会是我们第一次看到父亲躺在棺材里的样子。我感到很害怕，不想待在那儿。我深深地爱着我的父亲，看到他在棺材里毫无生息的样子，简直令人恐惧到无法注视。那样的情景不仅给我们带来畏惧，还有混乱。我不想去面对失去父亲的事实。当最后我看见他躺在那里时，我失声痛哭了起来，充满悲伤、悔恨和自责。我的胸口很沉痛，我的丈夫紧抱着我，拉住我，不让我倒下去。一想到以后再也不能和父亲聊天，再也不能照顾父亲，这样的事实让我无法想象，让我向它妥协是多么困难的事。我无法逃避这样的事实：他不再活着了，我再也看不见他了，再也不能和他聊天了，他就在棺材里，他已经过世了。

在计划为父亲守灵和举办葬礼的过程中，我和我的兄长们都很混乱，我们该告诉我们的亲戚朋友们什么呢？我们害怕被审判，当被问起父亲的死因时我们应该怎么回答？我们甚至会被认为是不孝、不关心父亲到何种地步的儿女，而父亲自杀是因为我们，他的孩子们没有尽全力照顾他吗？我非常害怕，害怕许多不知情的人会妄下定论。每当这时，我不想也根本没有精力去应对这样的问题。经过商量，我们一致决定保守父亲自杀身亡的秘密，没有必要把这件事情告诉每个人。

当在为守灵做准备并且尽力弄懂所发生的一切的同时，我的一个亲戚，不知从哪里得知了父亲自杀的事实，给我打了电话，她不是来安慰我的，而是开始指责我没有照顾好父亲。她因为父亲自杀的事埋怨我。我很吃惊，不知所措，感到非常不舒服。她让我遭受的痛苦超过了我能忍受的范围，我感觉被人重击心脏，深深的内疚和悲伤折磨着我。她的反应肯定和加深了我曾有的害怕——作为活下来的人，不管是公开还是暗地里被评论。这让我更加坚定要保守父亲因自杀而去世的秘密。

守灵

在灵堂上，我待在离父亲棺材非常近的地方。我想在还能见得到他的时候和他一起度过剩下的时光。看着他在棺材里毫无生息的躯体，唤起了我强烈的无法用言语表达的痛苦记忆。那是我过去从未体验过的巨大的悲伤。

每晚的守灵仪式结束后，朋友们各自回家，我也神劳形瘁地回家去。我犹如行尸走肉般，吃不下东西，也难以入睡。在家人的强迫下，我仅吃了一点食物。我变得消瘦，但这都不是我关注的事情。

父亲去世后的两天，当我从另一场守灵仪式结束后回到家，我的眼泪如洪水闸被打开一样，一哭不可收拾。我不停地大哭了三个多小时，一股来自内心深处的悲伤喷涌而出，无法掩盖和忍受。我的丈夫坐在我身旁，紧紧地抱着我。记得那天晚上，一想起父亲自杀而亡，我的眼泪就不停地流。到黎明时，眼泪早已流光，这时再也没有眼泪可流，也难以入眠，我只是感觉到一阵阵持续不断的头痛。

灵堂上出现的亲戚朋友们想知道父亲是怎么死的，他们的问题让我很难堪。尽管家里人决定了不再提及父亲自杀的事实，但是我觉得，关于父亲的离世不应以谎言覆盖，但又不能告诉他们事情的真相。所以，无论他们问了什么问题，我都保持沉默，因为我找不到一个合适的理由回答。

最后的告别

父亲的葬礼让人感到特别辛酸和痛苦。牧师安慰我们：死亡并不是生命的结束。他对我们说道，父亲到了天堂，一个远比人世间舒服的地方。在那里，他再也不会彻夜不眠，再也没有眼泪和恐惧。他已从痛苦中解脱，不再被束缚在尘世间躯体的无力和哀痛中，他来到上帝面前享乐了，总有一天我们会再次相遇。

这安慰简直不起作用，但我需要去聆听它。我需要一份保证，保证父亲在一个安全的地方，保证某一天我能再看见他。这让我坚持了下来，就像在坎坷的日子里找到一个平静的地方。但这个保证在葬礼仪式中并没有减轻我的悲伤。生理死亡是最终的和不可逆转的。整场葬礼仪式，表明从今以后，我和父亲要阴阳分隔了。

在整个仪式中，当我一回忆起父亲生活的点滴，尽管眼泪决堤而下，我仍努力设法保持清醒镇定。父亲作为一个单亲，为了撑起整个家庭，是多么辛苦啊。我知道，我会想念他的，想念我们在一起的时光。

在棺材运送到火葬场的途中，我回忆起和父亲在新加坡和国外的很多次旅行。想到这是他最后一次在世间的旅程，我很伤心。现在，他孤独地离世了，没有一个他爱的人陪伴着他，也没有我在他即将会到达的天堂。我知道，我即将面临的这场旅程是艰难的，但是无路可退。

第二章
当爱让我们受伤

父亲的遗物

父亲自杀而死这一让人崩溃的回忆似乎没有尽头。在葬礼之后的两三天，全家人到父亲生前所住的公寓整理他的遗物，令人忧愁的记忆又占据我的心头。

父亲的房间看起来和他活着的时候没有什么不同。房间里的一切都没有发生变化，唯一变化的是他走了，永远也不会回来了。我坐在他的床边，紧抱他的枕头。我努力地回忆起我曾与他度过的最后的那些日子，回想那段回忆是怎么样的，回忆父亲是什么样子的。我真的不想忘记，也害怕会忘记，然而当记忆如洪水般涌入脑海时，我又觉得它们极度折磨我。

他的每一件遗物都无情地提醒着我：他已经永远地离开了，他永远也不会回来了。那个他曾经用了很多年的杯子依旧有着父亲最爱喝的饮料斑渍。那些衣服，包括那件穿去教堂的最好的礼服，都整整齐齐地挂在他的衣柜里。当我在清理他的衣柜时，我惊讶地发现原来父亲是一个十分爱整洁的人。他的每一件衣服都挂得有条不紊。看到那件我多年前买给他的毛衣时，我哭了。这是他最喜爱的毛衣，因为它能让他感到温暖，尤其是在他晚年时。

当他的身体状况开始恶化、变得越来越虚弱的时候，他大部分时间都在这个房间里度过。这是他度过白天黑夜的地方，这是他度过日日夜夜的地方，然而对他来说，这地方并不安宁；这不是一个休息的好地方，因为他很劳累，在他生命的最后一段日子里失眠折磨着他；这是他吃饭的地方，自从他虚弱得到饭厅这么短的距离都无法行走的时候，他只能在这里进食；这是他梳洗的地方，因为他太累了，连走到浴室的路程都觉得像一场旅行一样。究竟最后他是怎样想方设法地靠自己挪到房间的那个窗户的呢？又是如何用尽全力地爬上窗台的呢？

他的轮椅，一件他非常鄙视的随身物品，放在了房间的角落里，再没有被动过。我们想尽办法让他坐在轮椅上活动，是为了帮助他更灵活些，但却遭到了他的抗议。这把轮椅很快就变成了他健康状况下降、丧失独立活动能力的标志。这把轮椅沉重地打击了他的自尊心，只有在极少数的情况下，他才勉强同意用它。相比坐在轮椅上被推出去活动，他宁愿留在这个安静的空间。

我环顾父亲房间时，看到了那台老式耐用的电视机。曾经一度在他的身体状况较好的时候，他会有足够的兴趣支撑着在床上坐起来，看他最喜欢的电视节目。自从他患上失眠症和妄想症后，他就对一切事物失去了兴趣，就连他最喜欢的电视节目——戏剧也不例外。如同这轮椅一样，这台电视也仅是房间里多余的一件家具。现在，它又似乎在提醒我他再也不需要用它了。

我的视线定格在父亲的日历上了。这是一种老式的、可撕的日历，每一页都会写上一个大大的日期。即使是在他最后的时间里，父亲还是很注意及时更新他的日历。直到他死的那一天为止，每天每一页都会被如期撕掉。这一天是停留在日历上的最后一天，仿佛时间就停止在他跳下去的那一天。

我极不情愿地整理着他的遗物：一大堆照片、纪念品和其他一些他积累了很多年的小玩意。这些照片中有他年轻时候的照片，那时他理了一个很时髦的发型，我直盯着照片上的那个人很久很久，心里很难受。不知为何，我情愿他回到我们的生活中。那一刻，我所恳求的只是希望他能够回来，这样我们就可以像往常一样谈话了。我想听他一遍又一遍地讲述他的故事，即使是不断地重复的，我也不介意。我只是想他回来，我愿意用所有一切做交易，只为让他重新活过来。父亲以自杀的方式结束生命，这个不可逃避的事实让我的丧亲和盼望之痛愈发强烈。他已经自杀了，这一直压抑在我的脑海里，说不出来。我极度需要再有一次机会来重写他的生命结束方式,他结束生命的方式本应该或本可以是不一样的。我无助地坐在那里,意识到自己对已发生的一切无能为力。

我的任务是筛选父亲的遗物,决定哪些该保留,哪些该舍弃。骤然发现我接受不了扔掉父亲的任何一件遗物,扔掉他的物品,就如同彻底摧毁他存在过的痕迹。这些是父亲遗留下来的一切,我想维持这一切,好让他能在我记忆中停留得更长久些。在父亲离去后,这里的每一件物品都变得如此珍贵。我想把他的所有遗物都带回家,但是理智告诉我必须舍弃部分,因此我挑选了一些物品,然后把它们整理入箱。我挑选了一些父亲在最后那段日子里所穿的衣物,这些衣物还残留着他最喜爱的肥皂的香味。我带走了父亲年轻时候的一些照片和一摞书,还拿了父亲的闹钟和手表。不管怎么样,这些与时间有关的物品是很重要的,因为我和他在一起的时光就在他爬上窗台的那一瞬间结束了。

我正要离开时,再次回头,希望看到父亲在门口送我离开——这是他保持了好多年的习惯。无论他多么劳累,多么虚弱,即使不得不使用他的助行架,他都会坚持目送我离开。当我最后一次回头看时,他不再在那和我挥手告别,多么残酷的现实啊。我带着装有他生前物品的小箱子,心中带着莫大的悲伤离开了他的公寓。

在开车回家的路上,我脑海中的一切都是关于父亲的点滴:想到他自杀了,我多么想念这位抚养我长大的模范父亲啊!如果他不是一位好父亲,也许我就不会那么想念他,自然也不会承受着这样的剧痛了。驾车回家的路勾起了我痛苦的回忆,曾经父亲就坐在我车的副驾驶座上。我一路开着车,逐渐地意识到,我再也没有机会载父亲了。我从前没有意识到,他在车上的陪伴竟是如此让我感到满足、幸福和安全。当我想到我再也不能享受到父亲的陪伴时,我泣不成声。

回到家,我把装有父亲遗物的箱子放进了书房。每次当我走进书房,我马上就想到了父亲,仅仅因为他的东西就在那里。我要守住那仅有的一点点联系。但是它同样也会引起我强烈的悲伤。最后,我决定把这个箱子放在一个不显眼的地方,一个当我想重温与他的记忆就能去的地方,一个当我感情脆弱时就能回避的地方。

回望与困扰

每一天，每小时，每分钟，只要我不想其他事情的时候，宿命般的那天所发生的事就会一直在我的脑海里回放。我哭了，想到父亲，也想到现在的自己。一旦有空闲，我的思绪就会飘到父亲那里去，想到他自杀的这件事情。回忆起驾车去父亲公寓的那个早晨和我们之间的最后一次谈话。每每如是，即便我不想记起，但我几乎能听到自己在那天和他说再见，和他那句令人怀念的"好的"。我想知道为什么自己没有发现他那次的回应异于往常。通常当我和父亲说再见时，他不仅会说"好的"，还会叮嘱我开车要小心，提醒我不要超速，总是让我注意饮食，饮食要规律，因为他知道我饱受胃痛之苦。为什么我就没有注意到这个简短而又忧伤的回答呢？

我发现自己一直在数着日子，感到时间过得太快了。我希望时间能够停下来，如果可以的话，希望能把我带回到他还活着的那天，那个父亲依然活着的日子，这样我能尽一切努力阻止他结束自己的生命。我希望时光能够倒流，能回到那段我能够把睡着的他抱起的日子。这样我还可以喂他吃饭，和他聊天，告诉他我很在意他，并让他确信自己不会孤独，即使他正经历着巨大的痛苦。

当我孤单一人的时候，关于父亲的各种思绪就变得格外清晰，格外形象。我不断被那些没有答案的冷酷问题困扰着。为什么父亲会自杀呢？在跳下去之前他在想什么呢？最后一刻他在想什么呢？那通哥哥打来告诉我父亲自杀身亡的电话不断出现在我的脑海里，我不禁感到震惊和内疚。我无法停止斥责自己为何没有多一丝警觉，为何没有看出父亲的痛苦，没有采取更多的措施。那天为什么我不待久一点？没有任何事情比在那天下午保全他的生命更重要了。为什么我不和他聊久一点？在父亲自杀之前的那天，保姆跟我汇报过父亲的情况：尽管父亲身体虚弱，精神也很脆弱，但他仍坚持走遍公寓的所有窗户。为什么我没有意识到这些情况的重要性呢？事后才明白，很明显地，他是在选择自杀的地点。

内疚与悔恨

当我想到自己辜负了父亲，我的心中就充满了内疚。我辜负了父亲，是我没有把他照顾好，保护好，也没有让他能够在晚年活得快乐些。如果他晚年过得快乐些，他就能安宁地回到天堂。头脑中无止境地重复着无数的"本应该""本可以""要是"之类的沉思，反思这些不同的可选择的结局绝对是一件极度折磨人的事情，但我控制不了自己，只要我没有其他事情要忙时，脑海里全是那些"要是"的情节。

要是那天下午我一直陪他就好了，他就会一直活着；我的出现本可以阻止这场悲剧的发生，要是我能从他的声音里听出他绝望的程度是如此的深，那他就会一直活着；在我们的多次谈话中，他都提到了渴望上帝能带走他，他不想成为任何人的负担，要是我当时对他说，他在我的生命中是多么重要，我是多么需要他尽可能长久的陪伴，那他就会一直活着。我错误地相信，家庭源源不断的关心和爱能帮助他度过人生中沮丧的时光。当他提到想去天堂时，我知道他是认真的，但我并没有意识到他那么渴望结束生命，我真的没有意识到他那时正在计划自杀了。他曾经是一个积极向上的人，尽管他很沮丧，但我始终坚守着一种希望和信念，坚信他会走出人生的低谷，因为他总能很快地恢复状态。要是当初我让他搬来和我一起住就好了，那样我就可以多花点时间陪伴他了。也许这样做，能让他不再感到那么无助，也许就不会感到被忽视了。如果我能够减少工作量，就可以腾出更多时间陪他了，或许这样会振作他的精神，他可能也不会选择自杀。我过去忙于帮助别人，也许是我忽视了父亲。

要是他能够有足够的休息，他的情绪就不会那么低落。我本应该更加重视他对失眠症的抱怨，本应该给他更强的镇静剂。那时候我不情愿给他服用过多的镇静剂，唯恐他会用药过度。要是我没有那么讲究控制过量服药，也许他现在还活着。

因为心中内疚，我每周都去看看父亲的骨灰壁龛。我会顺道去花店挑选父亲最喜欢的花，然后去他的骨灰存放处。我先清理之前插在那里的花束，再把新鲜的花束插上。在插花过程中，我在脑海里就会跟父亲说一些话。我会告诉他家里的情况，尤其是孩子们在学校的进展情况。父亲一向为外孙们的学习成绩感到自豪，无论什么时候，孩子们只要能在主要考试中取得好成绩，他就会奖励他们红包，鼓励他们更努力学习。

到他壁龛的这段路，我脑海中不可避免地涌现与父亲有关的记忆，他是怎么结束生命的。几个月以来，我每周都会去壁龛那里看看。这是我减轻内疚和负担的一种方式，也是我与父亲从某种形式上保持联系的方式。我记得我怀念他会怀念到心痛的程度。

因为母亲的壁龛就在父亲的隔壁，赤裸裸的事实是我的父母都已经离世，并且永远不再回来了。我经常泪眼汪汪，心情沉重地离开这里。要是我再有一次机会，我会让这一切变得不同。可悲的是，我没有讨价还价的余地；再也不可能有第二次机会；死亡已是定局，再做任何事情都不能扭转它。

我经历了一段分析或者说是尝试弄清楚到底出了什么问题的时期。"为什么会发生这件事?""事情怎么变得这么糟糕?""本可以做哪些事情来阻止父亲自杀呢?"我熟悉所有这种"要是"的情节，然而，它们却没有让我得出满意的答案。当我极度需要一些有意义的、能确定的答案时，我开始责怪其他人，他们应该为父亲的自杀负责任。

让我情绪抵触的人和事

父亲的死亡让我生活中各种原本平常的事情以及日常事务都蒙上了阴影。各种景物和声音像变了味道似的，都能引发新一轮的悲伤。每当电话一响，我的心就呼呼跳。这让我回想起父亲打电话过来，其实就是为了和我好好地聊下天。在房子里，无论我走到哪个角落，那里都有他来过的记忆。开车经过曾带父亲走过的地方对我来说变得艰难。因为这一切似乎都不可避免，我发现自己经常低头盯着马路，泪流满面。开车对我而言就是不停流泪，我经常一边开一边哭。

有些让我情绪抵触的事我能够预料和尽量避开。在开始的那段时间，我十分痛苦地避开那家我过去常常带他去剪发的理发店。我不得不收起父亲在我家爱看的 DVD，也不忍去听那些歌（他最爱听的）。每当我看到和父亲晚年时年纪相仿的老人时，我的喉咙就会哽咽。这些都是我早就能够预料到的。

但是有一些让我情绪抵触的事完全出乎我的意料，连我自己也不知道自己会受到影响，直到我发现自己哭了。有一次，我到水产市场去买新鲜的鱼，那天鱼贩子问我为什么（这次）买那么小条的鱼。这是一个毫无冒犯之意而又实际的问题，因为以前每周买鱼我都会算上父亲的那一份。我哽咽了起来，不自觉地泪流满面，低声说声抱歉就匆忙离开了。

家人和朋友

对我来说父亲葬礼后的最初几个月是非常艰难的。对我的丈夫和孩子们来说，这同样是非常艰难的。我不想谈论父亲和他的死亡，因为我无法接受父亲已经自杀的现实。我试图压制自己消极的思想和悲伤的情绪，我告诉我自己，这样做是为了保护我的家人，使他们免受痛苦和悲伤的折磨。如果我把痛苦与悲伤释放出来，我将无法控制它们。

如果父亲是死于年老或疾病，那么回想起过去美好的回忆或许会好受些。然而，自杀死亡是不同的。在一个家庭中，谁又能预知和预防自杀呢？当这样的事情发生的时候，我毫无准备；当它发生后，我也不准备去谈论它。在很多时候，它几乎是不能言谈的。因为没有哪些言辞可以充分描述这件事的惊悚程度，损失的巨大程度和悲伤的程度。

我能做的就是哭泣，每天除了哭泣还是哭泣，不知道何时就会突然流泪。我的丈夫是一个敏感的男人，在我哭泣的时候，他经常不知道要说些什么好。他不知道怎么安慰我。值得欣慰的是，他从不强迫我说出来，而是将我紧紧抱住。有时候，我并不哭泣，但会变得一反常态，毫无耐心，情绪激动。我的丈夫默默地忍受我火爆的脾气。

孩子们也不能置身事外。他们很安静，在我面前就像在鸡蛋壳上走路那样，小心翼翼地。很多次，他们尝试让我振作起来，却多以失败告终。我知道，他们和我一样，都挣扎在内疚和悲伤之中。但我还没有准备好和他们谈论这个话题。我害怕他们可能问到的问题，害怕面对那些我回答不了的问题。我对"为什么"和"怎么样"这种问题感到特别的焦虑，我该怎么开口说他们外祖父的自杀？该怎么解释他为什么会自杀？我缺乏勇气和精力来面对这些问题并安慰家里的其他成员。所以，我让自己忙碌起来，用沉默来掩埋掉所有的悲伤。我坚信这不是谈论他死亡的时候，坚信我不应该因为谈论它而给家人带来悲伤。然而，家里人还是从我那里发现了端倪。

除了父亲自杀这件事，我们谈论一切其他事情。家人都熟练地避开这个话题。它就像是在房间里的一件摆设，每个人都看到了，但都假装它不存在。

愤怒和责怪

我几乎每日都在和愤怒做斗争，每一天我都控制不了那让我愤怒激动的情绪。这是我疗愈之旅中最艰难的挣扎。在我的脑海里，我知道父亲选择以自杀的方式脱离苦海并非任何人的错误，但这一理性思维被甩到了后面。我责备我的哥哥、保姆、医生，甚至是上帝。

我在生自己气的同时，也在生我两个哥哥的气，因为我认为他们忽视父亲，没有能够在父亲生病的时候提供合格的适当的照顾。我觉得他们没有足够重视父亲，没有给予他应得到的足够多的关怀。父亲为了我们，他的孩子们，付出了那么多，而在他最需要我们的时候，在他身体最虚弱的时候，我们却没有尽力照顾好他。我们一起所做的努力和他能活下来所需要的照顾相差那么远。但我不想大吵大闹，父亲也不想看到这样的情景。所以我必须压抑我的愤怒，维持着家庭团结的假象，不管表现得多么的表面。我尽可能地避免与我的哥哥们会面，因为我害怕自己的肢体语言会出卖我心中的愤怒，并把矛头指向他们。但与家人见面的场景是不可避免的，我不得不努力克制我真实的感受。在与哥哥们谈话的过程中，我小心翼翼地压制着情绪，尽可能地避开谈论父亲和他离世的话题。我没有足够的信心管理好我的情绪，我害怕任何关于父亲自杀的谈论，因为这会引起我的愤怒。我会愤怒到说出非常伤人的话，并且不公平地指责他们，这有可能把整个家庭弄得永远支离破碎。

我对那个保姆感到极度愤怒。在所有人当中，那天她是最能阻止悲剧发生的,因为她在现场,看守好父亲是她的职责。相反,当父亲跳下去的时候,她却在打盹。这个盹以父亲的生命作为代价,以我的父亲和我的家庭作为代价。父亲是在她的看护下去世的。如果她没有睡觉,也许父亲还活着。父亲自杀后,我无法和她说话。因为我知道,我没有办法控制自己不说气话。

我对诊断父亲病情的老年病学专家很生气,因为他没有采取更多措施来帮助父亲。因为他不会和父亲讲方言,他就转而和我们沟通。如果父亲能够从他那里得到直接的保证(保证他的病情能逐渐痊愈),也许那样就能够给予他足够的希望,让他的生活能够得到平衡。

有时候,我的气愤并不是具体的。矛头主要针对医疗保健机构。我责怪这个体系,病人用很长的时间等待就医,而会诊的时间却只有短短几分钟。在没有考虑到有的家庭连保护病人安全都有困难的情况下,就给了一大堆的建议和处方。每一个医疗服务机构都应有的同理心又在哪里?为什么医生和护士都不尝试找出真正困扰病人的原因,找出能提供一些安慰的方法呢?是我质问太多吗?我也在生整个社会的气,因为每个人对那些虚弱的长者毫不在意。

我非常生气,荒谬地感到被惹恼,以致迁怒于上帝。父亲一生都是基督教徒和上帝的拥护者。尽管在生命中艰难的时期,他依旧坚持这种信仰。上帝本应该阻止这场悲剧的发生。但是为什么他不呢?父亲到底做了什么才会这样的呢?或者是上帝在惩罚我吗?如果是这样,那么我到底做错了什么?

我是在生气父亲做了这个决定吗?但是我已经目睹了他的痛楚,我怎么可以生他的气呢?很多时候,我能够理解他。明显地,他已经撑到了他再也无法忍受这种痛苦的地步了。在一定程度上,我特别理解他渴望结束连药物和祈祷都无法消除的痛苦的。老实说,我不能因为父亲自杀结束生命而生他的气。但是有一段时间,我为他以这种让人难以承受的方式离开而痛楚,为我成为他自杀的遗属而感到很沮丧。父亲曾经也是一位自杀的遗属。他曾经亲身体验过一个遗属必须承受的内心的煎熬与痛楚。所以另一方面我又不能理解他为什么也选择自杀。难道他没有意识到这会使我成为他自杀的遗属,这会使我因为这种无法理解和未能减轻的丧亲之痛而挣扎吗？

我的本能让我压制情绪，冷静地应对这些困境。所以，要克制如此强烈的负面和不安的情绪，对我来说是极其难受的。我不知道还能做些什么来摆脱内心翻滚着的焦虑。我感觉自己已经失去了平衡，我不知道如何恢复以往的内心平衡。我不知道做什么来宽慰自己。因为我不能表达我的愤怒，我只能把它变为我内心深处黑色的忧伤。生活变得毫无意义。

我在孤独中找到了安慰。樟宜（Changi）和东海岸（East Coast）的沙滩便是我的避难营。愤怒的海浪冲击着沙滩，然后从海岸上退下去，这情景如同我内心的混乱。这样能使我得到安慰，却不能带走悲恸。

双重悲剧

我的悲痛之旅因掺杂着多年前发生的事情而变得复杂了。父亲的自杀唤起了当年母亲去世时我的一些想法和感觉，这些感觉我不能也不知如何表达。正如你所知道的，我的母亲也是自杀的。那时我还在读小学，也不大记得当时的感受了。但现在，四十年以后，在失去父亲的悲痛时刻，之前的丧母之痛又回来了。

表面上看，我的家看起来相当普通，有父亲、母亲、两个哥哥和我。但是母亲还活着的时候，生活却一点也不正常。印象最深刻的是她是一个非常疲倦的女人，一个形存神亡的女人。她有相当长的一段时间幽闭在房间里，或者只是呆呆地盯着窗户外面。很明显，她是服用了药物，这使她变得嗜睡。当她醒来时，她看起来精神游离，健忘和消极。在我看来，母亲没有打算和我接触或者了解我。她沉浸在自己的世界里，我感觉自己被忽视。我不知道那时她正遭受抑郁症的折磨。

我想要一个能够像我邻居那样的不一样的母亲。她会煮饭，会清洁，会照顾好家人。我家是父亲承担了这样的责任。无论他多忙，我能感受到，他一直都陪伴在孩子身边，陪伴着他的儿子们，尤其陪伴着我。他会照顾我们的需要，陪着我们经历成长路上的身体上的疼痛和情感上的问题。这些本来是母亲的工作，但她却没有做。

另外，他也不得不照顾经常进医院的母亲，因为她屡次试图自杀。那些时候，他会跟我们解释母亲为什么去医院，是因为他没办法让她醒过来。每当这种事发生，我就会一个人留在家里，因为他要在医院陪着她。我很厌恨这样的事情发生，我不能理解母亲为什么经常想要自杀。但是我记得我的那种害怕、手足无措和被她抛弃的感觉，我还担心不得不在医院和家之间来回奔波的父亲。

母亲多次寻死，最终过量服药自杀。她在床上睡了整整一下午，父亲没能把她叫醒。我听见父亲一遍又一遍地叫她的名字，但她动也不动。我看见她面对墙壁躺着。父亲一定是叫了救护车，我记不起之后发生了什么事。但这一次她再也不能从医院回来了，父亲跟我们解释母亲因为服药过量死了。

我记不起失去母亲有没有特别伤心，因为我更关心父亲的安宁生活。母亲自杀而死，这给父亲带来了极大的悲伤和痛苦。我看见他哭了，这令我感到害怕。没有人给我解释过悲痛是什么，所以，我用孩子的思维推断出，眼泪是软弱和无能的标志。在葬礼上，我确保自己一直要陪在他身边，提醒他不再哭泣。我已经失去了母亲，不能再冒失去父亲的风险。我要让他坚强起来，我记得在母亲自杀的几周后，父亲问了很多"要是……就会……""如果……就好……"的问题。我认真地听着，虽然我不知道他到底在经受着什么。我所知道的就是我要提高警觉，不让他太悲伤，不让悲伤把他从我身边带走。我关注着他的情绪，在他看起来孤独时，我陪伴着他。我用我稚嫩的双手做家务活，以给他一些安慰。而我的兄弟们则在外面忙自己的活动。

父亲的存在让我有了一个孩童所需的安全感。因为我和母亲的关系不大亲密，所以在她死后的几年里，我没有真正地想念她。只有当我到青少年时，我才感觉到一种缺失。事实上，我没有想念她本人，而是非常渴望一位母亲的存在。无论他多么努力，依旧无法取代母亲的角色。例如，我意识到我身体上的变化时，却不知道向谁寻求建议和安慰，因为我是家里的唯一女性，我的月经初潮到来时，我完全没有准备。父亲不得不请求隔壁的女士来教我如何处理。我的朋友和同学似乎都很快乐，无忧无虑，适应得很好。我把他们的幸福归于他们有健在的双亲来指导他们，我觉得自己不如他们。我很羡慕我的朋友们，很生母亲的气，因为她没有能陪着我，因为我有缺失感和自卑感。但我又觉得这样生她的气很不好：毕竟她那时候患病了。

不知怎样的，我就跌跌撞撞度过了我的青春期。但是当我自己成为母亲后，这种缺失感又回来了。我再一次发现，自己在成为母亲这个关键点上，不得不在有经验的人的指导下应付这一切。我羡慕我的朋友们，她们的母亲会在她们坐月子的时候陪伴在身边，会为她们熬制产妇的食物，帮忙照顾孩子，这样她们就可以休息。我为自己感到遗憾，因为我要自行设法完成所有的事情，我是一个没有母亲的母亲。

很久以后，在我三十多岁的时候，我真正开始想念母亲，一个在我童年死去的人，而不是概念上的母亲。那时我已经读了一些关于抑郁症的书，甚至遇到一些患有抑郁症的朋友，所以我开始明白了一些她曾经一定面临过的挑战。我仍旧为自己感到遗憾，同样我也开始为她感到遗憾。我们相同的处境让我开始同情她。我的母亲是一个全职妈妈，她有三个孩子。在没有任何佣人的帮助下，她要自己应对这一切。如今，我也同样变成一个有三个孩子的全职妈妈，即便有佣人的帮忙，我还经常感到快要支撑不住，感到疲惫和孤独。

回头看看，我希望我能更多地了解她。我渴望听她谈论她自己，我想知道她想什么，感觉怎样，忍受着什么。我希望我们之间保持我所珍惜的母女关系。我没有一直惦记着她自杀的事，因为它似乎太久远了，和现在没有什么关联，直到父亲也自杀身亡。

在我为父亲感到悲痛时，我越来越意识到母亲自杀这件事加重了我被抛弃的感觉。为什么上帝允许我的父母以这种方式了结生命？为什么是我的家人？为什么是我？为什么？

耻辱与羞愧

如果我的父亲是死于疾病或衰老，我就会毫不犹豫地把这个消息告知我的亲朋好友们。但是在这个社会上，自杀被认为是一种耻辱，是很难被抹掉的。我发现自己不可能对别人的想法无动于衷。和其他遗属一样，我也需要面子。

在父亲去世以前，我对自杀的理解是肤浅的。我不能理解人为什么要以这种方式了结生命呢？是的，生活很艰辛，但是谁的生活何尝不是这样呢？我认为，那些选择自杀的人选择了一条容易脱离苦海的路。他们的借口缺乏说服力，他们是自私的，以自我为中心的。他们没有考虑到他们所爱的人会经历的痛苦，我相信其他人也会持有这样的观点，这就导致我要把父亲自杀这事保密。我不想其他人因为这样而贬低他。

我也为父亲因自杀而非死于疾病、衰老或者甚至是事故而感到羞愧。那位在灵堂上指责我没有照顾好父亲的亲戚，让我确信我会被其他人审判，无论是在跟前还是在背后，亲友们会认为父亲是因为感到忽视和不被关爱才自杀的。我将要名誉扫地，我也不想人们这样贬低我。

父亲自杀所带来的耻辱和羞愧让我很难为自己提供和寻求帮助。我属于社区中教会的一员。社区教会给它的会众提供支持，但是我却不能和牧师或者教友来讨论父亲的自杀。相反，我远离他们，保守着这个耻辱的秘密。我担心开诚布公只会引起他们的鄙视、躲闪、带有成见的好奇心和其他消极的反应。至多，有一些会同情我，会出于教会的互助互爱的责任而帮助我。但是我不想成为一个被同情的、让他们负责任的对象。

同样地，我也在远离我的朋友，避免看见那些令人失望的反应。每当我想要向她们吐露心声时，我满脑子都是想着她们可能会问的问题，还想着我会改变我现在的想法。我该怎么解释我的关爱和照顾还不足以让父亲不顾痛苦继续活下去呢？她们又怎么能明白我已经尽了最大的努力，但是却无法让父亲选择活下去呢？我都不能理解父亲为什么会选择自杀，更不用说向别人解释了。

考虑到父亲年事已高，朋友们一般都只认为父亲是衰老死亡的。我没有故意撒谎，但是也没有做任何事情来纠正他们的猜想。尽管那样，人们的敏感度之弱令我很惊讶。他们会很快地尝试安慰我，说父亲已经活得足够老了，没有什么可伤心的。其他人会对一些没有意义的平常话和吊唁滔滔不绝。我变得善于伪装成我可以处理得很好，我微笑着，大方地接受他们的吊唁。由于我的秘密的缘故，我所得到的支持，仅来自那几个暗地里地知道事实的朋友。我装作很冷静，很好地控制住自己的情绪，我感觉自己像个骗子。即使是出于好意，她们有时也会漫不经心地表达一些没有帮助的意见。她们当中有些人试图用他们伴侣或孩子也是自杀而亡的事来安慰我，这让我感到耻辱。很明显地，他们认为，比起他们在生命的黄金时期里失去伴侣，或是失去代表着自己未来的孩子来说，我父亲年老体弱而自杀身亡，我所遭受的悲痛可怕程度算少的了。因此，大家都觉得我不应该悲痛太久或太多，这样的推理模式完全忽视我与父亲的亲密关系。

无助和绝望

每天清晨醒来，我就会很想知道我应该做什么才能把悲伤埋藏起来。父亲活着的时候，他的需求会花费我大量的精力和时间。带他去看医生，到市场购买日用品是我的日常家务事。父亲很突然地走了。因为他的去世，我的时间富裕起来，想念父亲，想起他自杀那些时刻。当我想到我的内心有一个除父亲外别人都无法填补的位置时，当我想到自己到底要怎样继续活着时，一种深深的恐惧袭上心头。

生命怎么会变得如此脆弱和短暂呢？早上他还活着，眨眼间，下午他就离开了人世。在那么短时间里，生命就被扼杀了。在开始的几个月，我的生活失去了意义。我觉得他的死亡已经夺去了我生活的乐趣。没有乐趣，就没有希望；没有希望，生命就变得毫无意义。似乎每一天对我来说都没有什么盼头，我对自己处于万般无奈的处境感到很无助和绝望。如果生命只是充满了强烈的悲伤和精神上的折磨，那么活着的意义在哪里？然而生命还是要继续。心情很低落，感觉很糟糕，每天清晨我都难以振作起来。

好几个晚上我都梦到父亲生前的时光。我已经忘记了大部分的梦境，大概是因为我不想回忆，因为回忆会给我带来新的悲痛。但是有一个特别深刻的梦深深地印在我的记忆中，父亲问我为什么那么久没有跟他说话。这个梦是如此的真实。我非常难受，从梦中惊醒了，然后开始哭泣。

在戴孝的头三个月，我感觉自己快垮掉了。在很多场合，我一想到父亲或者谈论到父亲，就会突然大哭，我发现自己从神秘兮兮的忧伤突然会变得勃然大怒。很多次，我特别不理智地对待身边的人。或许他们对我的关爱可以让我感到很安全，可以让我宣泄我的沮丧、我的痛苦，但却无法减轻我内心的恐惧。我的家人仍然需要我来照顾他们的日常起居，可是，又有谁来照顾我呢？

第三章

谁帮了我？

　　失去父亲后，我多么盼望生活能回到过去，能逐渐恢复正常。即使父亲自杀这件事情已经过去了三个月，我发现情况并没有好转。庆幸的是生活上我还是能尽妻子的本分，妥当地料理日常家务，照顾丈夫和孩子们的起居饮食，甚至参加一些社区教会的教徒活动，继续参与救济院的工作等。慢慢地我感觉越来越力不从心，我控制不住自己的情绪，时常会情不自禁地大哭起来。我会在开车时哭，在家里哭，在大街上哭，和蒂娜在餐厅倾诉时哭，在教堂做礼拜时哭。无论我去哪儿，我总会想起父亲：和他去过的地方，一起进餐的地方，他看事物的方式还有他告诉我的事情。每当回忆泛滥，眼泪便会决堤。哭也许是一件好事，可以舒缓我的悲伤，但它是暂时性的，平静过后不久，我又会因为压抑而无法控制自己的眼泪。我感到疲惫不堪，已经失去勇气面对生活。大部分时间我是孤独和空虚的。在向蒂娜倾诉完之后我意识到要做点什么去改变这种生活。我不能再这样下去了。

　　蒂娜也是同样的意思，她温和地劝我向新加坡的援人协会（SOS）求助。她听说这个组织不仅帮助那些有自杀倾向的人，同时还服务自杀者的遗属们。

寻求帮助

　　开始的时候，基于个人原先的偏见，我拒绝了她的建议。我曾经认为咨询辅导是为那些需要并且有心理疾病的人服务的。在我眼中，那些人爱抱怨和爱烦躁，他们无法好好生活，还需要别人告诉他们该怎样生活。我不能想象为什么一个人会向陌生人寻求帮助来解决他自身的困惑。为什么这个陌生人可以做的家人或者朋友就不可以做呢? 我觉得我是一个身心平衡的人, 对我来说应对这些都不太难, 因为我有一个支持我的家庭和朋友圈子。可能这样的想法听起来让人觉得可怕, 但咨询辅导确实让我退缩。所以对于我来说, 所有关于我需要咨询辅导帮助的主意都是荒诞的。

在我印象中, 那些打 SOS 热线的人都有些类似的问题。一方面, 我同情他们, 因为他们身处困境, 也一定有极大的需要, 否则也不会和陌生人在电话里谈论他们的问题。我觉得这些打电话来求助的人是孤独和寂寞的, 他们没有什么亲人和朋友可以倾诉。另一方面, 我又想知道为什么他们不发展和维护家庭和朋友关系。如果他们这样做的话, 也就没那么需要打 SOS 热线, 把自己交给陌生人了。

虽然说是这么说, 但那时我还是不知道如何处理这些复杂的感情。我的丈夫和孩子们默默地支持着我, 他们总会在我需要陪伴或者空间的时候给我帮助。但是我不能够告诉他们我内心深处的感受, 因为我不想让我内心灰暗的想法影响他们。我不想让他们担心。蒂娜是我的好朋友, 她每天都会给我发短信或打电话, 每个星期我们都会一起吃午餐, 有时候还聊到傍晚 5 点。慢慢地我可以越来越自由地向她坦露, 但是我也担心每次聊天的焦点都在我和我的需要上会让她感到压抑。她一再向我保证她不会厌烦听我诉说我的悲伤, 反而是我厌倦了自己反复向别人唠叨自己的处境。另外, 她是我最好的朋友, 也熟悉我家的情况, 但很多时候当我需要客观建议时, 她很难做到公正。后来, 她想到了一个办法, 就是建议我去见见治疗师。我开始认真地考虑这事。我们在后来的几次午餐上还谈论了这事。

我也知道向治疗师寻求帮助对我来说也会大有益处, 他们能够比较客观地分析父亲自杀的事情, 从而让我能宽慰些。这会比随意向一个陌生人倾诉有效得多。但那需要我毫无保留地说出我的故事和想法, 以确保他们了解后做出客观的分析。蒂娜向我们保证, 我所说的他们都会保密。我也觉得向熟悉和专门服务于自杀家庭遗属的专业人员咨询或许会有效果。正如蒂娜所说的, 如果治疗无效, 我可以随时退出, 对我又没有什么损失, 试试又何妨。

于是我还是决定了要寻求这个组织的帮助, 但是要实施起来并不简单。某个工作日，我独自一人在家，拿起电话，然后就犹豫了。一直以来我都是以帮助别人的身份出现，想不到如今我居然要作为一个求助者去寻求帮助，这真的让人感觉很无奈。考虑一段时间之后，我还是一个键一个键慢慢地拨打过去，即使在那个时候，我仍在左右摇摆，不知道自己的决定是否正确。好几次，我拿起电话拨到一半又停了下来，不知道在电话里该怎么说才好。有两次电话通了，我努力地准备去和他们通话，但是最终还是没出声就挂掉了，我还没有准备好怎么开口。直到第五次，我终于开口了，先是了解了疗愈桥这个专门为遗属提供支持服务的组织。之后，接电话的工作人员让我稍等，她们要找负责这方面的咨询师来和我谈。

听到电话那头的那位女士说话，我很惊讶，她的声音是那么的和蔼、温暖。我放松了下来。她耐心详细地回答我的疑问，同时也询问了我何时开始成为遗属和我所失去的亲人等基本情况。她是那么的友好和善解人意，我感动得落泪了。在等待我恢复镇定的时候她沉默了，但即便沉默也不觉得尴尬。我决定了要接受她的邀请到 SOS（新加坡援人协会）去接受治疗。她似乎也觉察到了我的尴尬。在通话最后，我感到很舒畅。当然，我很乐意接受她的邀请去见她。这次的谈话给了我希望。我终于找到了一个专门帮助遗属的专家。我终于找到了一个我能够沟通的治疗师。后来我才知道，她是这个组织的首席执行官，她叫玛丽·马修。

一个疗程，两位咨询师

约好会面的日子越来越近，我变得紧张起来。我既没有被告知会谈时会发生什么，也不清楚要准备什么。我只是期待着见面，见到的玛丽会像第一次在电话里交谈的那端的声音一样温和吗？还是玛丽本人会和电话那端的声音大相径庭？如果不是蒂娜主动提出第一次会面陪我一同前往，我可能会临阵退缩。

我们来到了新加坡援人协会的黑色大门门口，按了铃铛。到这个专门为对生活绝望和有自杀倾向的人提供服务的地方让我感到很难为情。万一我碰到熟人该怎么办？他们会认为我也是有自杀倾向的人吗？还是认为我仅仅只是一个需要被帮助的人？来到新加坡援人协会，我不得不承认我是一个需要别人帮助的人。曾经的助人者现在变成了受助者，这让我感到羞愧和难堪。这也让我更加了解了求助者的心理。

我被带进了一个方形的房间，房间里有三张靠背椅和一张桌子，桌子上放有两份报纸和一些关于该组织介绍的小册子。房间是密闭没有窗户的，这样就没有任何人可以窥视偷听了。另外他们还端给我一杯暖暖的茶。直到今天，想起第一次和玛丽的会面，我仍不会忘记这杯茶带给我的温暖与舒适。

玛丽长得又高又瘦，看起来很和蔼可亲。很快我便开始讲起关于我父亲自杀的事情来。令人出乎意料的是，虽然叙述这件事情真的让我很痛苦难受，以致忍不住流泪，但我却在她的支持下敞开心扉谈论我的故事，而且我感到很舒适。遇见她，我就像找到一个知己，她的陪伴让我可以毫无防备地讲述自己的故事，从第一次见面开始，直到之后的几个月里，我都切实地感受到安慰。我不再感到孤独，因为在这里有人能够理解我，能够通过问些引导性的问题，好让我能更容易地讲述我的故事。最开始那种与陌生人见面的疑虑和不安都已消失殆尽。于是，我同意继续接下来的会谈。

在第二次会谈中，当我在讲述失去父亲的痛苦时，玛丽也忍不住落泪了，我被深深地感动了。玛丽的眼泪表达着她对我的理解，并且像是在告诉我她愿意和我一起经历这段艰难的旅程。她娴熟敏感地运用会谈的技巧，引导我一步步叙述当天所发生的一切，从而帮助我疗愈。玛丽像外科医生一样，慢慢地用刀切开我的伤口，排干伤口里的脓液。伤疤被揭真的很痛。但她从没有让我带着敞开的伤口回家。相反，她用仁慈、关怀、温暖、同理甚至眼泪，慢慢地缝合我的伤口。那一刻像温和的镇痛软膏涂抹在被感染的伤口上一样，帮助伤口痊愈。

即便如此，每次会面时我都会大哭一场，回家后也颇觉头痛难忍。我记得每次回到家，我都需要睡觉休息才可以缓冲过来。我们约好每两周会面一次，但有时我并不想去赴会，因为每次会面都需要回忆起那段刻骨铭心的时光，相当折磨。相反地，用忙碌来逃避显得容易得多。有很多朋友想和我一起用午餐，有很多杂事需要处理，还有很多家务需要做，还有我的丈夫和孩子需要照顾……这一切都给了我借口，连两个星期一次，一次就一个小时的会谈我也没时间参加。讽刺的是，我是找到了能够倾诉的人，但我总是想方设法去回避那些议题，因为那样比向蒂娜倾诉更痛苦。我知道，如果我一直推迟治疗的话，我需要更长时间才能痊愈。尽管咨询辅导让我感到身心疲惫，但我还是觉得治疗是有效的，毕竟它让我不会像以前那么悲观绝望了。在玛丽给予我的专业治疗下，我对生活重新有了希望，也感受到一切都在逐渐恢复和好转。和玛丽的会谈是我疗愈路上实实在在走出的一步。

最终，玛丽只给我做过四次辅导。在第三次会谈时，我看到她坐下和站起来都有点困难。她的背受伤了，尽管如此，在咨询辅导过程中她还是努力地听我诉说。我记得我还提醒她多注意背部，平时要小心慢慢地坐下和站起来。她在我们第四次会面后就住院了。不久后，工作人员告知我要取消我和玛丽的下次会面了。我没想到从那之后她再也不会回来了，或许连她自己也没想到。十个月后，即我父亲自杀后的一年零一个月，玛丽就因为癌症去世了。我是在《海峡时报》上得知她去世的消息的。

带着极度沉重的心情，我参加了她的葬礼。那里有许多和我一样在她的协助下走出或正尝试走出哀痛阴影的受助对象。大家一起唱圣歌歌颂她的一生，我不由自主地想起了一年前父亲的葬礼。她的死对我来说是另一个沉重的打击，我走到墓碑前追忆她，不自觉地也哀悼我那自杀身亡的双亲。我不明白上帝为何要如此善良的人遭遇这种痛苦，以至他们不顾别人能否帮助他们，自行了结生命。伤心的回忆不断涌现，我不敢继续参加她的火葬礼仪，因为我怕这一切会唤起我的伤痛回忆。于是，我提前离开了。我们短暂的相遇给我留下了不可磨灭的印象，她是新加坡援人协会里相当不错的一位助人者，是她给了我足够的勇气，让我以遗属的角色步入丧失至亲之痛的疗愈旅程。她在我最需要帮助的时候雪中送炭，深深地感动着我。感谢上帝让我遇见了她。

在玛丽住院休病假期间，我被告知会有人来接替她的工作和我进行会谈。我十分不愿意接受这样的提议。我觉得无人能代替她，何况我也不想重新再向别人讲述我的故事，那是何等的沉重痛苦。我不能确定接手的治疗师是否够专业，我心里面充满了疑虑。她会像玛丽一样温和仁慈吗？会是一个很好的倾听者吗？她有能力让我很好地表达出最近的感受么？那时我在想，或许是到了停止接受治疗和新加坡援人协会说再见的时候了。我告诉自己，我与玛丽的四次会谈治疗已经足够让我走出阴影恢复正常生活了，我要独自面对接下来的人生。向玛丽敞开心扉，之后又突然间失去她，让我感到很受伤。我不想再次经历这样的事情了。但遗憾的是，我连报答玛丽的机会都没有。那是一份永远偿还不了的人情债。

我告诉自己要控制好自己的情绪不让自己悲伤，让所有的痛苦都过去，无论如何也要跨过去这个坎，只要让自己忙起来，我就能好起来。忙碌将是一种万能药。我开始尽可能地让自己忙碌起来，甚至忙到没有时间让自己愧疚的程度。确保每时每刻都有工作、社会活动或其他活动等要处理。首先，一天我要做我三个女儿的司机，多次接送他们；期间，和朋友一起吃早午餐和喝下午茶，并且参加许多教堂和救济院的志愿工作。我奔波在每个活动中，使自己没有任何闲暇想起那折磨人的一切。我努力压抑着自己的感受，就像将自己的想法和身体剥离一样。但这反而让我感觉更不好。无缘无故地我很快又压抑起来，害怕面对任何事情。我的情况越来越差。我知道我需要专业的治疗来帮助我。于是我带着抗拒的心理拨通了代替玛丽的那位咨询师的电话。

奥菲利娅和玛丽很不一样，以至于开始会面的时候有些困难。玛丽安静和婉约的性情和我有点相似，在接受会谈辅导以外的时间里，我们还一起喝咖啡，仿佛我们俩是朋友一样。但是奥菲利娅显得更活泼外向一些。在我讲述我的故事时，她的身体会向前倾并且会配合手部肢体语言强调她在提问。她需要更努力些才能引起我的配合和反应，只因我仍想着玛丽，不情愿重新投入另外一段咨询关系中。开始的时候我也拒绝向她讲述关于最近作为一位遗属的故事，因为那样仿佛在重新揭我的伤疤。但奥菲利娅和我都坚持了下来。最终，在一年半的时间里，我们总共做了三十次会谈。

奥菲利娅和玛丽的咨询辅导方式完全不同。玛丽是温柔细心的类型，而奥菲利娅则是不拘小节。玛丽擅长捕捉我分享故事的细节，甚至在我们的某次会面中，玛丽就谈及了这些小细节，让我感觉像是和老朋友在交谈一样。奥菲利娅则更主动活跃，她回答我所提出的各种具有挑战性的问题，并且引导我自己去寻找答案。甚至有时，奥菲利娅会故意问我一些没有答案的问题，但这些问题提升了我对自己作为一名遗属的认识和感受。我不知道什么时候问题会出现，因为她在思考问题的时候，总会皱起眉头来。随着我们接触越来越多，我开始信任她，并从中得到安慰，慢慢地开始盼望和她的会谈。我也发现我们都会用类比或暗语的手法来讲述事情。有时她还会用笔和纸画出我们谈论的事物，让我越来越能理解作为遗属所经历的悲伤。现在，我已经习惯她的开放且直率的会谈方式，并从中得到安慰。

我描述和比较两位咨询师并不是要告诉大家哪个更好，只是想强调她们在我生命中的重要性和解释清楚我为什么需要治疗。我不知道认识她们是我的幸运还是我的不幸。如果可以的话，我不打算认识她们和向她们寻求帮助。但是同时我也认为能和她们交朋友自己很幸运。她们由内而外表现出来的同情心、责任心和爱心让我不断有勇气面对父亲自杀的创伤。毋庸置疑，我来新加坡援人协会接受治疗这个决定是正确的。

在接受新加坡援人协会的辅导中，我学习到了每位遗属都是独一无二的。每个人都有自己悲痛的故事，处理这些创伤的方法也没有对错之分。我们各自都有让自己恢复和重建生活的方法。对我有用的未必对下一位接受辅导的遗属有帮助。但在新加坡援人协会这里，确实有些东西能够帮助到我。

隐喻治疗法

在一次会谈中，我谈到我的愤怒、愧疚、失望、伤心和困惑。我感到我的这些负面情绪像羊毛球那样混乱地纠缠在一块，五味杂陈，让我感到很无助。有些感受我甚至都不知道该怎么形容它们，还有对能说出来的感受我也不知所措。然而现实生活中，我是一个生活有规律的人。我习惯安排整理好生活当中各种各样的事情，包括我自己的感受和情绪。譬如我在家里用完某样东西后都会把它放回原处。但是现在我感觉整个人都很混乱。奥菲利娅建议我一件一件事情慢慢来，每次处理好一件事情。这个主意听起来很简单，但它却真的让我有信心控制好这些混乱的情绪。我从这样的类推中领会到，尽管会很痛苦，但我能在帮助下一次处理好一种负面情绪。

后来，她问道，假如有一天我自己解开了这些纠缠在一起的思绪我会怎么办? 这样的问题让我很惊讶。我开始问自己，难道一直以来都是我在作茧自缚吗? 这个比喻让我开始明白我其实可以用好的心态来面对发生在我身上"坏"的事情。这让我感到震惊。我意识到虽然我不能控制任何事情的发生，但我可以根据自己的生活经验和策略来面对和处理这些事情。这也提醒了我要对自己有耐心，康复是需要时间的。

治疗中，我们一直用这样的一个比喻: 有一位遗属，他被带到一个陌生的地方，被强迫去完成一段旅程。然而对我来说，这怎能让我不害怕呢? 尤其是要我独自去完成这样一段未知之旅。因为我知道冒险本来就具有许多的不确定性。虽然我不知道走完这段旅程需要多长时间，也不确定最终能否走出这个地方。但至少我知道这肯定是一段精彩的旅程，有时感到不安也是很正常的。这个比喻让我豁然开朗。难怪之前自己感到那么茫然不知所措和无助了。我也逐渐能够用这样的比喻来帮助我回看作为遗属的这段经历。这在开始的时候具有挑战性，也挺吓人: 不知道自己身在何方，也不知道往前自己会面对什么。对我来说，真的很难想象有一天我会开始好起来。但是在我得到新加坡援人协会的帮助之后，一切显得没有那么艰难了。自从父亲自杀后，我第一次感到轻松，也重新看到了希望。后来，我参加了专门支持遗属的小组，我感到很安慰，那里有很多和我一样的同伴，他们或是已经度过了困难走到了前面，或是还在后面，又或是正和我一起经历这段疗愈悲伤的旅程。

在我哀叹父亲没有能够得到善终时，我会用隐喻的办法来治疗我的这种伤痛。对我来说，他是一个称职的父亲，但是为何他要以悲剧的方式来结束自己的人生呢? 奥菲利娅问我如果把父亲的一生写成一本书我会分成多少章节，每一章节该怎么写? 我想用 10 个章节来描述他勤恳、称职、奉献和忙碌的一生，以有点悲惨的第 11 章记叙他最后的时光。我喜欢这种方式的隐喻治疗，因为它让我突然明白在我和父亲的生命故事里还有 10 章是那么美好。我可以自由地选择任何一个章节去阅读或者去重读。父亲在我记忆里永远是那么的美好，我没必要困在第 11 章，没必要困在那些不开心的情景中。

我对这种隐喻治疗法很难忘，因为在辅导中，还有在我感觉低落的时候，它都给了我支持。

哭吧、哭吧不是罪

去接受咨询治疗意味着要去讲述失去父亲的痛苦，还有每次都哭泣着结束治疗。眼泪也是疗愈的一部分，或者说它是必要的一部分。但如果您只是抽泣或者哀号，那么眼泪和疗愈之间并没有明显的关系。在我的认知里，哭泣是疗愈良药的这种说法和我开始时的经历并不相符。从某些方面来讲，哭泣可以让我们得到安慰，因为它释放了痛苦。但（这种释放）并没有让我感觉自己在好起来。相反地，我感到精疲力竭、崩溃和害怕，觉得自己再也不能振作起来。让人尴尬的是——还要在一个陌生人面前哭泣。这打破了我平时的给别人以安慰，整洁而优雅的女性形象。

哭泣让我感到虚脱和头痛，在每次艰难的会谈后，我都不得不大睡一觉才能够缓和过来。我曾经无数次想过要放弃所有的咨询，因为它与我的期望不一样，事实咨询上反而让我变得更加糟糕。只是我仍相信咨询师提醒过我糟糕之后就会好起来。每次会谈结束前她都明确告诉我："每次来看我之后你可能会感觉更糟糕。"她是对的。所以我学会了调整我自己的期望。我相信一切终究会好起来的，相信眼泪会冲刷掉我的悲伤和痛苦。同时我发现，我很久没有在外面哭过了，因为眼泪都在咨询室流干了。

在家里，我只有在不会引起太多注意的情况下偷偷哭泣，尽可能地避免在孩子们面前哭。我也尝试在会见要好的朋友时控制住自己的眼泪，虽然很少能成功。但是在新加坡援人协会这里，只要我愿意，我可以尽情地放声大哭。在我的咨询师面前哭泣，意味着我可以得到关怀和安慰，同时也避免了给家人造成困扰。随着时间的推移，哭泣成了疗愈的一部分。逐渐地，我的哭泣变得没有那么激烈了，人也感到轻松多了。

笑吧、笑吧不是罪

笑也是治疗的一部分。可能大家很难想象笑和自杀哀伤辅导会有怎样的关联，但是幽默确实在其中扮演了重要的角色。笑在生理上可以产生胺多酚，一种由身体产生的神经递质，能有效地消除痛苦，可使人不需要借助人造物质（药物、酒精、食物等）达到兴奋状态。我的咨询师总能谨慎和敏感地运用她的幽默感。

以前我总喜欢笑。你别看我个子小小的，我可爱笑了。然而，在我父亲自杀之后我就没有笑过了。我甚至认为，笑是不对的，笑或者是快乐会显得我不够爱我的父亲。我应该一直默哀，证明我对父亲的爱不是肤浅和短暂的。但是会谈时奥菲利娅总能让我放声大笑，而且我不会感到愧疚，甚至还有点开心。她还将我们的私人笑话记录在我的康复治疗记录手册上。她还开玩笑地说记录在表格上以便更好地追踪我的康复日程。当意识到这很荒唐，我不由笑了起来。曾经我还将我的康复日程表看作股票市场走势图。

有时候，不是奥菲利娅故意逗我笑，而是不知不觉我就会笑起来。记得有一次会谈，我抱怨说每到周六我都会感到特别难受，因为以往每周六我都会花上整天时间陪伴父亲，而现在他不在了。奥菲利娅听后说我的一个星期里有七天：星期一、星期二、星期三、星期四、星期五、伤心日、星期日。"星期六"被她艺术化地说成了"伤心日"①，我不由笑了起来。我认为笑是一种释放，让我从父亲自杀的阴影中解脱出来，让我顿悟了一些我曾经同别人一样不理解的事情。在认同把星期六命名为伤心日的过程中，我尝试允许自己在星期六尽情悲伤，我不期望别人懂得我的周六，毕竟那只是属于我的而不是其他人的周六。

当我能重新笑起来时，我也变得更容易宽恕自己了。奥菲利娅常常调侃我的控制欲。从某种程度而言，这帮助我认清了一些事情。当然，我本来可以更好地照顾父亲，但是现在不管我多么努力地控制局面，天堂这一边也永远不可能完美如初了。我也慢慢地明白到父亲也不希望我失去微笑。所以我努力让自己时刻保持兴奋，哪怕是小小的冒失，也可以让我开怀大笑。

---

① 原文 Saturdays 和 Saddays 音相近

偶尔生气也没关系

前几个月我一直压抑着自己内心的愤怒，而现在它却以我始料未及的方式爆发了。我迁怒于花园里的杂草，而以前我一直认为园艺的乐趣在于无须抬手就可以欣赏花的美丽，感受花草的气息。父亲自杀后，我铲光了那里的花草来发泄。但这并不够，我还需要其他的发泄出口。很快一个银行的办公职员就倒霉了，因为发现一个金融产品有问题我便肆无忌惮地破口大骂，当时所有在银行的人都看着我。这件事情破坏了我的形象。那是我人生中第一次在公共场合那样做。

我在咨询会谈时也会毫无缘故地愤怒生气。过了一会，当我冷静下来后，我想知道我究竟是为什么生气呢？原来我是在为自己需要依赖咨询师来弥补自我内心失去的东西而生气。我觉得很不舒服，尤其在我觉得她帮助我只不过是她工作的需要，而不是因为她真正想帮助我。我想要约她会谈也是有限制的。我是多么的希望当我有需要的时候我就能够拿起电话打给她啊，但这是不可能的，因为她辅导我的时间越长，从专业角度来说，她就越不被允许和我成为朋友，那个我随时都可以联系的朋友。父母先后自杀让我更加的敏感，觉得自己被他们抛弃了，而心理治疗师没能在她的工作时间外帮助我，这也让我生气。

我也会因为奥菲利娅对我的叙述的回应感到生气。很多次，当我说到心痛难受，哭得稀里哗啦的时候，她却看起来很平静，不为所动。她尽力同理我的感受，但是在那个房间里，我觉得只有我一个人受伤，这让我很生气。

我们还会反复谈到我对兄弟们的恼怒。最后，奥菲利娅问道："假如你不给机会让自己去原谅你的兄弟们，对你来说这以后将会是怎样的呢？"

我吃了一惊，对她很失望，因为她给了一个我不想要的建议，我焦躁沮丧地离开了咨询室。第二天我打电话跟她抱怨。她认真听了，之后还对不能很好地理解我的情绪表示抱歉，我也原谅了她。

在临终关怀医院做志愿服务的过程中，我有幸读到伊丽莎白·库伯勒·罗斯写的《论死亡与面对死亡》[①] 一书，了解到悲伤有五个阶段，但我没想到愤怒会这样让人觉得不舒服和不可理喻。然而，为了疗愈康复，我需要让自己理解和学会表达愤怒。

絮叨一下也无所谓

我觉得我非常需要向奥菲利娅一遍又一遍地讲述我父亲的故事。蒂娜也是我重复哀悼和追忆父亲的聆听者。但我并不会向家里人说太多，因为这是我能做到的保护他们的一件事情，何况他们让我开心起来已经很不容易了，我不想因为我自己的沉思而让他们失望。

蒂娜见过我的父亲和家人，和她追忆往事会容易些。但是这也有局限，即便是最亲密的朋友，她一个人又能够帮我分担多少呢。我更愿意和我的咨询师去分享，因为她是专业的聆听者，我不至于会对她造成困扰。大多数时候都是我在回忆和父亲一起的时光，讲述他为我们子女奉献一切。当然我也会说一些想念、哀悼或者生他气的话。只是我会有所克制，因为我怕她会觉得无聊冗长。所以在她问到的事情上我才会说。我很感激她在会谈时总会问我同样的问题，以便我一次又一次地追忆父亲。

其实我并不太想回忆父亲的事，但我还是要讲。我能很有条理地讲述故事，感觉别人在和我一起承担，我的痛苦也就没有那么沉重了。同时讲述也让我明白到我尽到了做女儿的责任。我的心理压力稍有减轻，我的痛苦也减轻了许多。和聆听遗属故事的专业咨询师分享是百利而无一害的。她告诉我讲述是非常重要和不可或缺的。所以我对她一遍又一遍地讲，直到我不再想要倾诉。

康复的过程并不是一条康庄大道

开始咨询时，我想如果我用心地参加每次会谈，我就会进步。我曾经渴望康复的过程会像一条直线那样，一开始会伤心，但最终会康复治愈。

①　On Death and Dying，Elizabeth Kubler Ross（伊丽莎白·库伯勒·罗斯）著

我希望每完成一次会谈我的悲伤就能减少一些，经过一系列的会谈我就可以回归到我本来的正常生活。我想尽快走出悲痛的阴影，早日摆脱对心理咨询的依赖，继续自己的生活，因此我很看重治疗的速度和进展。我甚至还打算和家人一起移民，开始崭新的生活。我想离开这，到新的环境，这样伤心的回忆才会渐渐淡去。

然而我发现只有我是那样想的。奥菲利娅曾告诉我，每次见完她之后不一定会变好，有可能会感到更糟糕。事实也是如此。我情绪总是先坏透之后才会慢慢地好起来。虽然如此，我仍坚持自己的治疗进程时间表。经过一年的咨询后，我觉得是时候和她说再见了。所以，在我们之后的一次会谈时，我握住奥菲利娅的手，感谢她。接着我又主动捐款给新加坡援人协会以回馈他们对我的帮助。

仅仅在两个星期后，我再次打电话给新加坡援人协会，请求会谈。我发觉自己更加压抑，需要更多的辅导会谈。对我来说，再次回到新加坡援人协会是一种挫折，但很遗憾我又病了。这次奥菲利娅提醒了我和父亲之间的父女关系很紧密。他是我一生中最重要的一个人，我怎么可能那么轻而易举地将父亲自杀的事情放下呢？要问我认识他多少年了？整整47年。你说这需要多长时间去忘怀呢？我曾经以为用一年的时间去康复和治疗已经够长了，而我认识父亲一辈子了，我想我永远没法翻过这一页。我移民只是离开和他一块生活的熟悉的环境而已——我还是会时常想起关于他的伤心往事。那时候我又怎么面对那些痛苦的刻骨铭心的回忆呢？可以仅仅将回忆留在新加坡吗？很显然我只能继续接受康复治疗。正因为深爱着父亲，所以他的离去让我十分痛苦。如果我以远离这个伤心之地来摆脱痛苦，这对我与父亲的感情来说很不公平。我爱戴我的父亲，只要想起他我都会感觉伤心难过。我想如果我只是尝试用距离来进入忘却的阶段，这对于父亲来说也太不公平了吧！

慢慢地我意识到我的生活已经不可能和从前一样，再也不可能回到过去的正常轨道，而我需要调整心态重新适应新的生活。生活发生了改变，不仅仅指我的父亲已不在人世，还意味着父亲自杀后我的经历和感受也改变了已有的生活。

悲伤的过程循环反复，一次又一次地触碰同样的问题、感觉、想法和回忆。有时候这些强烈的感觉会淡去，但是很快又会恢复。我变得期待这种感觉回来，尤其是在喜庆的节日里。没有父亲在的第一个圣诞节我感觉特别的难过。我敏锐地感到他的不在场，也没有心情庆祝。以往圣诞节都在我家举行，每次我都很盼望大家的到来。但是这次我却不能过好这个圣诞节，会想起父亲已经永远离开了我。但我记得父亲总想要所有孩子聚在一块庆祝节日，所以我还是带着沉重的心情去庆祝这个节日，只是我总感觉有点悲伤，总感觉还少了点什么。我只知道自己的悲伤情绪和周围美丽的装饰和欢快的颂歌格格不入。以前圣诞节后，我们还会一起过中国的新年。在圣诞节来临前，我发现自己非常想念父亲，我的心里满是期盼，但随后又极度沮丧，但这种感觉不再困扰我。有时候我心里仍会感到愤怒，甚至明显地表现出来，只是没有以往的那么强烈。我知道我不会再有像以前那么强烈的感觉了。

当我不再刻意处理那份悲伤时，我发现自己开始能够更好地接受和拥抱现实。当我不再刻意将它驱逐出我的心里时，悲伤也不再完全侵蚀我的心灵，让我有更多的空间去回忆美好的东西。因为自杀，我失去了父亲，这成了我生命中的一部分，不管我去到哪里或者做什么，这是不可能改变的事实。同时父亲温和、慈爱的形象也深深地印在了我的脑海里。①

---

① 作为译者，对这段文章最大的感受是，对于有过创伤的人来说，我们不是要刻意地去处理所有的痛苦，有些伤痛是忘不掉也撇不开的，刻意的处理反而让我们更加痛苦。我们应该要学会安顿它，安顿内心那个受伤的小孩，只有这样，我们才能有更多的空间去接纳更美好的自己。

第四章

何去何从？

父亲自杀后，我花了一年多的时间参加由新加坡援人协会专门为（在生活中经历打击的）遗属开展的支持性小组——疗愈桥，并在小组成员的相互理解和支持中受益。尽管在我第一次致电新加坡援人协会的时候就问过"疗愈桥"，但这只不过是我开始接受会谈的一种方式。直到我开始写这一章节的时候我才逐渐明白。其实我并没有想过要参加支持性小组，我想其他遗属也体会过我所说的最初的那种不情愿。

踏上疗愈之桥

虽然玛丽曾经告诉我"疗愈桥"这个平台能让我坦露自己内心的挣扎，还能让我得到其他有类似经历的人的支持，但我死活也不愿意参加。我视自己的隐私为至上，只有少数亲密的朋友知道我父母自杀的事，甚至我的牧师和教会社区的教友也不知道那些细节。因此，我真的不能想象自己跟一群陌生人分享自己的隐私是什么样子，和一个陌生人——新加坡援人协会的治疗师分享已经如此艰难了，我没法想象把自己的伤口挖出来让这么多人看会是怎样的。

在父亲自杀前，我并不了解支持性小组。每次在书本或电视节目上看到，我以为就是一群人围成一个圈坐下，分享想法，并由最大声的那个人来主导整个分享。他们似乎情感空虚，每周重复地分享他们各自的戏剧般的故事，也没有具体的目标。我根本不想参加这样的小组。

同时，我很怕在"疗愈桥"碰上熟人。我担心在那里说的话会传出去，那样的话我需要作很多解释——父亲的自杀并不是由于我对他的忽视,但这似乎更像是我为自己辩护。

我似乎没有必要参加支持性小组,我有蒂娜,而且我已经从玛丽还有之后的奥菲利娅的辅导中得到很好的支持。她们都在我想见她们的时候,慷慨地安排时间和我见面会谈。她们也从来都不会强迫我参加支持小组。

我写到这里才忽然意识到,我不愿意加入到"疗愈桥"的另一个主要的原因是我的自尊心在作祟。我还记得童年时父亲做生意失败,我们不得不依靠别人的接济过活,后来更是被迫搬到更便宜的住所,那也是母亲的抑郁症刚有苗头的时候。刚开始那段艰难的日子里,我对需要依赖别人产生了恐惧感。因此,后来我甚至极其厌恶要找专业治疗师治疗的想法。

事后反思,那时我害怕与别人分享自己的经历会不可避免地带来负面情绪。或者更糟糕的是,我会因为其他遗属分享的故事感到更加痛苦。他们的亲人自杀的故事会给我带来更多难以承受的悲伤和痛苦。总是想起父亲自杀这个不开心的事情是毫无意义的,我要做的就是把它忘记。

那么,我是怎样完成"疗愈桥"的疗程的呢?事情的转折点出现在父亲去世周年纪念日之后的几个月。在多次终止治疗和移民计划失败之后,我重新接受了辅导。但不同的是,我对其他遗属是如何处理他们的情绪和生活产生了强烈的兴趣。他们的内心也同样饱受内疚和愤怒的煎熬吗?他们也在同样痛苦和期盼中徘徊不前吗?我多么希望我不是唯一一位在亲人自杀一年后还难以走出痛苦阴影的人。特别是在节日里,如亲人忌日、生日还有圣诞节和春节等家庭聚会的节日里,他们是如何度过的?我很想知道他们是不是也对这些场景感到恐惧。我也不像一年前了,我已经做好了与其他遗属见面并且聆听他们经历的准备了。

我的治疗师告诉我,在小组中也有一位组员的父母自杀逝世的。我就想他肯定能明白我所经受的,不然还有谁能体会到双亲都自杀离去的痛苦呢?也许在那些遗属当中,没有谁真正能体会到在至亲自杀很久后,仍然在痛苦中挣扎的感受。奥菲利娅可以让我理解自己的经历和感受,但她毕竟没有这样不幸的经历,因此无论她怎样换位思考,她都无法体会我的痛苦。

我还有一个困扰,我怕我的那些好友们已经厌倦听我的反反复复地跟她们倾诉同样的事情。而"疗愈桥"小组可以为我提供新的支持，因为我的悲伤需要更长的时间才能消去。

随着时间的推移，我不再那么害怕在"疗愈桥"的会谈中碰到熟人或朋友，也许这是因为我想得更明白了。既然"疗愈桥"只对遗属开放，那么他们肯定也对这一点有所顾虑。而且，在某种程度上，我的内心越来越强大，可以不去理会那些不理解我们的人的看法，或者说我至少觉得自己有勇气去尝试这样做。

另外，我加入"疗愈桥"小组还怀着一定的"救世主"的情结——我很希望到那里去帮助一些同样有需要的人。也许，这种方式能够让我尝试去理解我的父母亲为何自杀。我感到自己好多了，也想帮助其他刚遭受痛苦的遗属，希望对他们有用，那样的话我就不必总是接受别人的帮助了。因此，当奥菲利娅再次向我提起这个支持性小组的时候，我答应了。

第一次小组会谈

当我开车去参加第一次的"疗愈桥"会谈的时候，我很是彷徨。我想我会听到怎样的故事呢？那些故事又会对我产生怎样的影响？我很害怕父亲自杀的情景重现，我会被悲伤包围。我感到很孤独，也很后悔没有叫上蒂娜来陪我。尽管到现在为止，我已经无数次去过新加坡援人协会接受个案会谈，但这次又是一个全新的开始。每次驾车经过那个 U 形的标志，我都有一股掉头回去的冲动。车外的雨下得很大，又碰巧遇上了堵车，这个完美的借口让我打电话告诉新加坡援人协会的办公室说我去不了了。我紧紧抓住方向盘来加强前进的决心。我到达新加坡援人协会的办公楼时，花了一些时间停车，鼓足了勇气走进入口，甚至在按响门铃前在门外还踌躇了好一会儿。一位工作人员打开门把我引领进去。这时，已经开弓没有回头箭了。

在正式见到其他遗属之前，我就听到了她们的笑声。我怀着忧虑的心情走了进去，以为会是一种严肃甚至是低沉消极的氛围。她们的笑声似乎有点不合时宜，在如此严肃的场合，我可笑不出来。

我被引到新加坡援人协会办公室的培训侧厅，那也是"疗愈桥"小组的会谈室。奥菲利娅和两位遗属在里面，当奥菲利娅向她们介绍我时，她们上前逐一和我握手。利安和乔安妮的丈夫都是自杀离去的，她们重新生活已经两年左右了。我印象最深刻的是她们俩没有自怨自艾，而是尽力像往常那样去生活。与其说她们在接受"疗愈桥"的康复治疗，倒不如说她们和援人协会的工作人员在会谈中相互促进。

我们边喝茶，吃吃点心，边等待其他人的到来，她们当中有失去了配偶的，有失去兄弟姐妹的，还有失去父母或孩子的。会谈开始，奥菲利娅提醒我们为了让大家安心分享自己的故事，我们应该对会谈的内容保密。当每个人分享自己的故事时，大家都哭了，或是为自己，或是为别人。作为独立的个体和作为因为亲人自杀而同样经受痛苦、能相互理解的一群人，我们努力地与伤痛做斗争。

当轮到我分享的时候，我感到一股又一股的悲伤涌上心头，同时也伴随着一点点的释放。我并没有抱着通过分享就能摆脱失去父母亲痛苦的想法和希望，因为我清晰地知道那种痛苦会伴随我的余生，或许在某时某刻它会变得更加强烈。在小组内，我跟他们的经历有很多相似之处，我可以很安心地分享我失去父母亲的痛苦，因为我们都是一样的，没有人会去评价或是谴责我。我不能跟我的家人谈论我的悲伤，因为我想让他们远离悲伤，不想让他们为我担心。作为小组的一员，我可以畅所欲言，这里的人能理解我的感受，并且让我有一种归属感。尽管我们来自不同的背景，拥有不同的信仰，但意外的是，第一次会谈之后，小组成员很快便形成了团体。开始我以为，因为我们之间的共同点，我们每个人的情况应该都会差不多。但是事实并非如此，每个人的情况都不一样，有些人要比别人更加消沉些。我需要对这个小组改观。满怀复杂的情绪，我们结束了第一次的会谈，让人欣慰的是，我觉得自己终于能和其他遗属聊天了。六次会谈后，我感到小组成员的感情联结得更强了。组员之间互相交换了电话号码，以便日后需要找人分享悲伤时可以联络。我收到了小组组员给我发的信息，说当我想要分享的时候可以联系他们，那种支持让我万分感激和感动。

自那以后，我在两年内参加了四个"疗愈桥"小组。每次都会有新的成员加入小组，每一个新进来的人都带着自己的伤痛故事。老组员通过分享引导新组员，老组员的出席对那些刚刚失去近亲的新组员来说就是一种安慰和力量。由此表明，老组员也是引导新组员走出困境的巨大力量。

遗属们

（在小组中①）谈论我的痛苦和失落，倾听每个新成员的故事，让我逐渐更能承受自己的悲伤，孤独感也减轻了许多。虽说奥菲利娅与我的个案会谈在我的疗愈过程中起了至关重要的作用，但在我不断好转的时候，她还得去辅导其他人。而我和其他遗属们的关系就不一样了，因为我们身上都有着共同点，这让我们成为真正的同行者。和他们一起的时候，我觉得我们的关系可以更深一层。我可以在自己觉得有需要找人倾诉的时候随时打电话给他们。我之前沉溺于痛苦的孤独感，此刻被这些故事所驱散。下面是一些让我记忆深刻的故事（为了保护他们的隐私，我修改了他们的真实名字以及个人信息）。

希拉的故事

希拉的母亲多年来承受着抑郁症的折磨，最后从他们公寓的走廊上跳楼结束了生命。因为和希拉有很多相似的境遇，我和她有种特别的亲近感。她年迈的母亲和我的父亲在同年同月以同样的方式结束了生命。同样地，希拉也是家里唯一的女孩，就像我和父亲一样，她和她母亲有着特殊的感情。希拉的母亲与抑郁症抗争的经历让我情不自禁地想起了我的母亲。听着希拉说起她母亲陷入昏睡并且对所有的活动都失去兴趣的时候，我逐渐明白我母亲那时都经历着什么。和希拉一起，我开始哀悼我的母亲，通过希拉的母亲抑郁症的故事，我开始理解我的母亲，而这种理解要比阅读任何一本关于抑郁症的书更透彻。

希拉在分享故事时显得非常悲伤，边说边流泪，听起来她已经极其疲惫。就像我一样，她那时正处于艰难的时候，在照顾自己的同时还得照顾

① 译者注

家人。在家里，她的孩子们不愿意看到她哭泣，因为那样会使他们感到不安。因此每当她落泪时，她那四个孩子就想安慰她，让她别哭，然后让她和他们一起玩。我能理解孩子们的做法，因为当年母亲自杀后，我也不让父亲哭泣，我担心父亲会被悲伤所淹没，甚至因此自杀。我紧紧地陪伴在父亲的身边，每当他伤心时，我就去安慰他或转移他的注意力。当我在小组中分享这部分故事时，我意识到我太早熟了，对一个小孩来说，对父母亲的安全负责这个担子实在太重了，可能这就是导致我这样的孩子从小开始多愁善感的原因吧。打开心扉，与组员分享我人生的插曲让我痛苦不堪，我记得我泪流满面地走出了会谈室，悲痛欲绝，作为一个小女孩的那段痛苦记忆让我背负太多了。我僵硬地在其他组员面前走过，奥菲利娅陪着我走出了会谈室，她的举动对我而言意义非凡，也让我更清楚地认识到，一直以来尽管极其痛苦，但我从来都不是一个人在战斗。现在回想起来，其实我没有必要走出会谈室，在其他组员面前哭泣也无伤大雅。

希拉还提到在她母亲自杀后，兄弟姐妹间的矛盾凸显。家庭不和加剧了她母亲自杀所带来的痛苦。我的家庭也一样，在父亲自杀后的几个月里，尽管我们兄弟姐妹之间没有公开的冲突，但至少我能感觉到我和我的兄弟们之间的关系是紧张的，我们之间的关系有了微妙的变化，再也回不到从前了。

我被希拉的疗愈历程启发和鼓舞了。在过去的一年里，希拉已经参加过一轮"疗愈桥"会谈。这是她参加第二轮"疗愈桥"的辅导会谈。虽然失去母亲的痛苦犹在，但她已经愿意坦露自己与这种痛苦做斗争的过程。虽然她还是很悲痛，她却安慰着旁边的组员。当我在她第三轮的"疗愈桥"辅导会谈中见到她的时候，我听到她把来新加坡援人协会参加"疗愈桥"小组比喻成"回家"。在这里，她可以毫无顾忌地和我们谈起她的母亲，她说我们就像她的家人一般。在某次会谈中，希拉戴着她母亲的金手镯过来，以前对她来说这是一件何等困难的事情，但现在却成为她和母亲保留一点联结的方式。

我被希拉鼓舞了，这让我有动力回去看看我哥哥的公寓，也就是我父亲度过余生的地方。至今为止，我仍然害怕再回到那公寓，害怕那些关于父亲最后那天的痛苦回忆再次涌现。自从收拾了父亲的一箱子遗物后我再也没有回去过，再次回去对我来说算是个里程碑。我直接回到了父亲的房间，他的床是空的，食橱也是空的。当我回想起父亲在他房间里的样子时，我哭了。随后，我进了客厅，父亲最爱的椅子还在，记得当父亲在这张桌子上吃饭时，我曾无数次坐在一旁陪在他身边。最后，我看了看父亲跳下去的那扇窗，我忍不住哭了。我再次回头看了一眼然后关上了公寓的大门，一切都结束了，那时，我终于战胜了我的恐惧。

乔安妮的遭遇

乔安妮在她的丈夫自杀后，用尽全力去重整自己的生活。她的丈夫在接受精神治疗之前已经被抑郁症折磨了好几个月，但治疗并没有使他的病情好转。在他们结婚周年纪念日那天，乔安妮接到女佣的紧急电话说她丈夫从卧室的窗户跳了下去，她急忙赶回家。

当我在"疗愈桥"遇到她时，她丈夫已经去世两年了。我第一次到"疗愈桥"接受会谈辅导时所听到的笑声就是她的。那时我并不知道在她的笑声背后还蕴含着她为了两个女儿继续勇敢坚强地生活的动人故事。每次听到她分享故事，我都能感觉到她有多么的孤独。一夜之间她便成了寡妇和单亲母亲，首先她得解决经济问题以及那些平常由她丈夫处理的琐事。更不幸的是，她的父母并不如她所料地支持她，甚至她的公公婆婆还责备她没有照顾好她的丈夫。她感觉自己被丈夫背叛和抛弃了。她曾尽自己所能去安抚和支持他，他明明说会坚持的，但为什么最后还是放弃了。她无法理解，他明明说爱她的，为什么却要离开她。

乔安妮对失去配偶最强烈的失落感莫过于当她带着孩子们出去的时候，看到别人一家子一起散步或吃东西，这个时候，她的小女儿（在她丈夫跳楼时，小女儿刚好在家）就会很伤心地问："为什么我没有父亲？"

当她的小女儿上小学时，班上的同学谈起他们的家庭时，她问乔安尼问得更加频繁了。

我很佩服乔安妮，特别是她那敢于跟组员吐露自己的经历和心声的勇气。她的语音语调甚至都能透露出她的想法。她参加小组对我们，特别是对新组员很有帮助，因为无论我们有多消沉和痛苦，她都能让我们安心地分享。同时，她让我们敢于说出自己消极的情绪。她也谈到她挣扎过，甚至有过自杀的念头。如果不是因为玛丽给她的精神支持的话，乔安妮自己或许都已经放弃生命，选择跳楼自杀了。玛丽是乔安妮的治疗师，也是后来在"疗愈桥"小组跟进乔安妮的，玛丽提醒乔安妮要为她的孩子活下去。

乔安妮的经历让我明白配偶的自杀会带来多大的痛苦。她说起的孤独感和被抛弃的感觉引起了其他有同样经历的人的共鸣。当我第一次听到她的故事的时候，我被她的坦诚触动了。她对丈夫离她而去、只剩下她独自照顾两个女儿表现出很愤怒。但最近，她的愤怒转移到一些难以处理的事情以及工作的压力上。她丈夫生前，无论何时她工作不顺心，只有他能察觉并安抚她，让她冷静。在他自杀后，他仍然是乔安妮泄愤的对象。

"当我心情好的时候，他可以很安静地待在那，"乔安妮说，"不然的话，我就会骂他或诅咒他。"

乔安妮说她再也开心不起来了，但她尽力让她的孩子们过得开心，哪怕是在一周疲倦的工作后，她也要带她们出去玩，也要在假期抽空陪她们。每次她和其他组员淘气地开玩笑时，她总会泪光闪烁。乔安妮对"疗愈桥"小组给予组员的支持坚信不疑，因为大家在一起相互分享经历。她始终相信我们能够通过小组的治疗康复过来。

雅辛塔的过去

雅辛塔唯一的儿子自杀了，她的经历让我沉思：在这世上没有比孩子自杀更让人痛苦的了。她的孩子是从街口的公寓跳下去的，那时他还在接受抑郁症治疗。那天，雅辛塔还煮了他最爱吃的饭菜等他回家，可惜他却再也回不来了。雅辛塔在她的儿子去世大概四个月后参加了"疗愈桥"小组，因此她悲伤的情绪还很强烈。当轮到她分享的时候，她再也忍不住了，泪水奔涌而出。在家里，她没法说起她的儿子，因为她的丈夫和两个成年的女儿并不愿意和她去谈论心中的失落。他们都知道雅辛塔正处于悲痛中，不想再增加她的痛苦。同样地，雅辛塔也一直抑制着不哭，保护着自己的女儿们，不想让她们悲伤。

雅辛塔为儿子的自杀感到很自责。她觉得，要是自己这个当妈的能做得更好的话，他可能就不会自杀了。家里的很多东西都让雅辛塔想起她儿子。看到他的拖鞋，雅辛塔就想他是不是还活着。有那么一瞬间，她甚至认为他可能并没有死。她没有动过他房间的任何东西，并经常躺在他的床上。当雅辛塔说到她会抱着他的枕头，闻着他的 T 恤留下的气息，努力地回忆一切关于儿子的故事的时候，我也和她一起哭了。她说到他戏弄她，还说起他和他的宠物猫以及玩枪的样子，每每这些都会勾起她痛苦不堪的回忆。儿子的猫对她来说既是一种安慰，又是一种痛苦的提醒。工作时，雅辛塔表现得很正常，但她一回到家就没有力气去做饭或做家务了。然而在儿子去世前，雅辛塔每天都起得很早做家务，准备好早饭后才去工作。如今她觉得很疲惫，因为在儿子死后她一直都睡不好。

第一个疗程的"疗愈桥"小组会谈结束，小组也解散了。四个月后，当我再次参加下一个疗程的"疗愈桥"小组时，我也没有见到雅辛塔。她的两个亲人去世了，她们家再次沉浸在悲痛中。但我至今还记得在小组最后一个会谈时雅辛塔给我们带来她焖的鸡肉，依然记得当我们称赞她的厨艺精湛时她所流露的笑容。

阿甘的经历

阿甘的弟弟在工作上遇到了一些问题。他开始变得很消沉，最后在街口的房子跳楼自杀。阿甘很生他弟弟的气，气他弟弟毫不考虑自己的自杀会给这个家庭带来多大的影响。

"就算他不考虑我这个哥哥的感受，他又怎能这样对待父母呢？"阿甘悲叹道。

阿甘来到"疗愈桥"后对抑郁症有了更深入的了解，他想弄清楚他弟弟自杀的原因。首先，他想学习防止其他家人自杀的技巧，他很懊悔没有更好地了解自己的弟弟。他弟弟很少与人交际，也从没有向家人倾诉过自己的心声。无论弟弟遇到什么麻烦事，他都是第一个去询问，只是弟弟往往没有任何反应。阿甘希望以后家人能更好地沟通，但家人之间的交流随着他弟弟自杀事件的发生而变得更糟糕。怀着学习的热情，阿甘准备阅读一些书籍，却发现在"疗愈桥"图书馆的书都是外国人撰写的，没有本国的遗属写过他们的经历，而我写这本书的部分原因正是想满足这个需求。

讲完后，阿甘哭了，阿甘在分享自己无助时的坦诚触动了我。当谈到自己没有救回弟弟以及不想悲剧在这个家庭再次发生时，阿甘落泪了。阿甘决心让他的家庭变得更美好，但作为遗属来说这将是一段很长的历程。我在想阿甘会不会走得太快了，我觉得他应该给自己更多的时间从失去弟弟的悲痛中走出来，然后再寻找解决问题的途径。

王氏夫妇的悲痛

在儿子自杀前，王氏夫妇没有注意到他们成年的小儿子已经身陷困境，所以小儿子的自杀让他们很震惊。在四个孩子中，小儿子是最让他们省心的，一直都很独立，可以照顾好自己。当我在"疗愈桥"小组遇到他们的时候，他们已经在这件事上抗争三年了。但对他们来说，就连想怎么去处理已故儿子的遗物都是件悲痛的事情。他们分享道，他们的好朋友和亲戚们常常劝他们："都已经过去那么久了，为什么还不放下往前走呢？"他们却难以做到，每次看到他们的侄子、同事的儿子或其他年轻人，他们总会想如果他们的儿子还活着的话那该会怎样。

王氏夫妇很努力地去面对永远失去儿子的事实。他们夫妻俩相互支撑，先后寻求过精神顾问和新加坡援人协会的治疗，他们也参加了"疗愈桥"小组。像其他和家人一起参加的组员一样，他们被安排在不同的小组，给他们各自的空间去分享自己的悲伤。在小组中，没有任何的约束，也不用担心自己的分享会给自己的家人带来影响；在小组中，他们可以尽情地宣泄自己的悲伤，组员们没有任何客套的安慰话。

我们没有任何的心理准备就得承受至亲自杀去世的事实，但那确确实实发生了，这让我们明白到什么是重要的，也让我们明白在经历过疲惫和恐惧，面对过困难后，我们仍拥有美好的回忆。

透支——我们都应该好好保重

在"疗愈桥"的小组会谈中，我注意到刚成为遗属的组员总比自杀事件过去久一点的组员看起来要更疲惫和消沉。他们看起来像没有睡好，眼睛没有神采并且黑眼圈很明显。他们背负着沉重的悲痛，身体也被压垮了。小组中有些组员谈到自己根本无法入睡，另一些组员说到感觉自己的身体不是这痛就是那痛，好像很容易就会病倒。然而他们却继续努力工作，让自己忙起来，以此来麻木自己。

在刚开始的时候我也曾如此，生活的点点滴滴都让我承受着巨大的压力，压得我的胸腔痛得无法呼吸。在开始的无数个夜晚，父亲的自杀一直困扰着我，让我无法入睡。我的身体很疲倦，但我需要去解决看起来比休息更重要的事情。我甚至故意让自己忙起来，参加各种活动，想去逃避悲伤，但那让我更累。我陷入了这种恶性循环当中，丝毫没有意识到那是我身心疲惫的源头。

那时我不觉得饿，也吃不下太多的东西。某天，我的朋友说我看起来非常憔悴，在浴室里称下体重，我竟然在几个月内瘦了三公斤。然而我都忽视这些自己身体疲倦的警告信号，因为我觉得自己过得很好。

在一次和咨询师奥菲利娅的会谈中，她说我花了很多的时间和精力致力于济贫院和教堂的公益活动。她建议我让自己慢下来，不要那么拼命。她还说在帮助别人之前先照顾好自己。我很礼貌地倾听她的话，但并没有重视，我甚至翻了下白眼（当然这只是在我的脑海里），因为我根本就是蔑视那种自我照顾的想法。对我来说，我身边人的需要才是最重要的，我可以做很多事去帮助减轻他们的痛苦。照顾自己就是自私的，就是以自我为中心的。我觉得我并不需要照顾自己特别是我可以合理安排自己的时间和完成所承担的义务，因此当我踏出会谈室时，奥菲利娅所说的话已被抛到九霄云外了。

对我来说，我很难接受自我照顾这个概念，因为从小到大我都在照顾别人。自从母亲自杀后，我就成了家里三个男人外的唯一的女生。从七岁起，我就开始帮父亲干家务活，也照顾着父亲。母亲自杀的事让亲戚们像躲霉运一样躲着我们, 父亲照顾着我们, 而我也照顾着父亲。数年后, 我去了国外念书, 我也不断地为来自世界各地的留学生在物质和精神上提供支持, 帮助他们安定下来。当我回到新加坡时, 我依然和他们保持着密切的联系。甚至在我处于忙碌的状态时, 我都会很自然地去照顾别人, 无论是在以前还工作的时候, 还是后来成为妻子和母亲时, 都没有改变过。

在长达七个月的会谈中, 我突然感到很担忧, 我才意识到照顾好自己的重要性, 不然的话真的好可怕。我不想借助药物去应对对未来的恐惧, 因此我还是接纳了奥菲利娅的建议——让自己慢下来。我暂时不参加济贫院的公益活动, 让自己能够休息, 同时也减少了提供朋友精神支持和联系教堂的时间, 把注意力放在自己身上, 给自己留点时间。这就意味着我有一段很闲暇的日子, 我也害怕消沉的思想会在脑海中挥之不去。为了避免那样, 我开始和朋友去散步, 或独自去散步; 我的胃口也逐渐好起来; 我开始涉猎休闲书籍或杂志, 还有一些小说或鼓舞人心的作品。奥菲利娅曾教我一些深呼吸的技巧, 每当我焦虑时都能奏效, 我停下手中的东西, 只关注自己的深呼吸, 这样就可以冷静下来。我开始写日记, 这样我可以在会谈中很坦诚地分享我日常的点点滴滴。

我花了很长的一段时间才明白, 处理悲伤并非易事。用忙碌来替代自我照顾只能在短时间内让我忘记悲伤, 让我麻木和暂时不想起父亲, 但这不能也不该是让我从悲伤中走出来的长久的良方。

恐惧也是正常的

我没有向朋友提过自己的恐惧, 但在父亲的葬礼后, 生活又回归到了正常的轨迹, 我时常感到孤独和害怕。我不断想着父亲的自杀, 以致不能控制那些思绪在头脑中萦绕, 我都觉得自己快要疯掉了。

当在"疗愈桥"小组听到其他组员分享他们也面临着恐惧时, 我释然了。实际上, 我们都有着各自具体的恐惧。约瑟夫恐高, 那是因为他的母亲从他的公寓跳了下去。每次从公寓的窗户往下看时他的腿都会发软, 而不得不扶着东西去支撑身体。没料到, 一个成年人也恐高。阿甘怕自己会再有家人自杀, 因此当他们之间出现问题时, 他总会引导着他们加强彼此的沟通。尼克提到他对药物的恐惧，在他父亲自杀后，他曾因为太悲痛而去看医生。处方上的药物虽然奏效，但尼克仍然恐惧药物，因为他父亲自杀前也是这样一直接受抑郁症治疗的。

我们就是这样，作为成年人去承认这些不合理的恐惧。当我听他们分享故事时，我意识到自己并非异类。对于遗属来说，我们并没有疯掉，即便有自己快要疯掉的想法那也是正常的。

隐私与保密

当我们经历过不幸后，学会的第一件事便是"戴着面具"，这是"疗愈桥"小组的一位组员提出的。周说（在妻子自杀后①）他和他的朋友们相处得很不开心，朋友们都避开他，因此他必须假装自己能应付得很好。他的朋友们不想听他一遍又一遍地复述他妻子的自杀。在他妻子自杀后，在守灵和葬礼上他们都给予了周精神上的支持，但他们希望周忘记过去重新开始。因此，每次和朋友出去，周就假装放下了。约瑟夫也一样，每次和同事在一起，除了母亲自杀这件事情，约瑟夫和他们无所不谈。失去了儿子的王氏夫妇，在家也假装一切正常以免让其他孩子和他们年迈的爷爷伤心。每当王氏夫妇感觉悲伤涌起要将他们淹没时，他们就会跑到外面去哭。

我们除了努力让痛楚远离自己的朋友和家人外，我们也戴上面具来保护自己不受别人的评价和审视。我猜想在亚洲的人际关系中，"面子"是如此的重要。尽管我感觉自己是一个开明的人，但仍觉得家人自杀是件让人羞愧的事，因此我瞒着很多人。我不停地提醒自己，父亲的自杀并非因为我。虽然我有时会显得没有耐心和不那么善解人意，但我已经尽了我最大的努力去照顾他。渐渐地，两年过去了，我终于有勇气告诉更多的朋友关于父亲去世的事实。但有时，我仍说父亲是死于年迈，撒谎让我坐立不安甚至内疚。我觉得我会对大多数人撒谎是考虑到他们没有必要了解真相，不是因为我还觉得羞愧，而是父亲自杀本来就是我们家共同保守的秘

---

① 译者注

密，基于尊重我家人的隐私权，我决定用笔名写这本书，以免引起别人对他们不必要的关注。但是，在小组分享时我用了自己真实的名字，我不知道我的哥哥们有没有对他们的朋友说起过父亲的自杀，在某种程度上我对此有过怀疑，但他们并不需要公开。

每当我看到媒体对自杀事件耸人听闻地进行报道时我都很愤怒，我很幸运没有被媒体报道，但是约瑟夫就没有那么幸运了。媒体追着他数周，直到他逃离家一段时间才肯罢休。

伤人的评论

有时候，在人们与遗属们交谈时，或许是无意的，但大家缺少思考的话语总会带着几分冷漠和麻木。亲戚、朋友或熟人的一些评论非但没有用，还会对当事人造成伤害。这样的话题不断在"疗愈桥"小组的会谈中出现。它影响了一批又一批新加入的和以前加入的遗属们。

我记得在父亲自杀后的某一天，在他的灵堂上，一个亲戚将父亲自杀归因为我没有把他接到我的家里去照顾。我极其受伤，因为她的意思是我需要为父亲的自杀负责任。她的话激起我的自责、内疚和悔恨。我冲进洗手间，哭了起来。

其他经历过不幸的人也同样被别人欠考虑的话折磨过。

一个失去儿子的组员曾听人这样说："至少你这样总比那些不见了孩子的人好多了。"

乔安妮的朋友对她说："已经过去那么久了，你为什么不改嫁呢？"

目睹王先生失去儿子半年后，他的老板劝导他说："我希望你不要再悲痛了，重新投入生活吧。"

开始的时候我以为他们只不过是一些局外人，并不理解，站着说话不腰疼罢了。但是，有些遗属们自己也会这么说。希拉的兄弟不忍看她哭泣，对她说："逝者长已矣，生者如斯夫，哭又能怎样？"

我的一位失去丈夫的熟人对我说："我失去丈夫比你失去父亲痛苦多了。"她不是"疗愈桥"小组的成员，万幸的是，我的小组其他组员没有说过这样让人难受的话。

有时候，一些话并没有想要伤人的意思，而仅仅是普通的节日问候，但对一个遗属来说，去回应"圣诞节快乐""新年快乐""生日快乐"的确很痛苦。正如乔安妮说的："有什么值得开心的？反正我再也开心不起来了。"

所以也就不奇怪为什么，有些人会像阿莲那样选择在节日出国，以逃避这些节日里的互相问候和家庭聚会，因为家人亲戚们相聚的情景，让阿莲对痛失丈夫的感觉更为强烈。

也许有时候，人们在交谈过程中只是不知道要说什么去打破沉默，所以说了些缺乏考虑的话。也许是因为他们不善于表达自己的意思。也可能是因为他们很恼火遗属不断地回忆逝者，跟他们抱怨不公。总有一些人不知出于什么原因和目的说这样的话，那些话加深了遗属们的痛苦。一些遗属故意躲开那些心思迟钝的人或忽视那些不懂得自己感受的人所说的话。我发现跟朋友聊聊自己听到的这些伤人的话能减轻我的痛苦。

在我和其他组员一起的疗愈历程中，最触动我心弦的是他们愿意真诚坦率地与大家分享他们的故事，在治疗自己的同时，也帮助他人从悲伤痛苦中走出来。是的，"疗愈桥"小组让我接触了很多悲伤的故事，但也让我对人类坚韧不屈的精神有了更深的认识。从这里我学到了：我们可以跨越悲伤，跨越痛楚。

第五章

上帝啊，您在哪儿？

我无法向您祈祷。

这不是我要的旅程。

是它选择了我，我无言以对。

噢！上帝啊！

您为何要这样将他带走？

我无法向您祈祷。

那震惊，那现实，

那让人震惊的现实。

噢！上帝啊！

您在哪？

当我父亲死去的那一天，您又在哪？

您让我如何向您祈祷？

就连我心中最后的一丝安慰您都要把它拿走。

是您，先让自杀带走了我的母亲；

噢！上帝啊！

您是不是觉得我从苦难中还学得不够多？

现在又以同样的方式带走了我的父亲。

您让我如何向您祈祷？

让我的悲伤成河。

剥夺了我的希望，让我伤痕累累。

噢！上帝啊！

您看到我的心在流血吗？

上帝啊！

我已疲倦不已。

茫茫人海中，我踽踽独行。

我需要您的帮助。

我的话语充满了愤怒，

但我脆弱的灵魂却充满了悲伤。

上帝啊！

您总该听到我的呼唤了吧，

又或只是我没有看见。

因为当我再次回首时，

我看到了您的恩典。

他们热情地伸出双臂，

紧紧地抱着我。

和我一起走过这段旅程

我们手拉着手一起走

尽管泪水成为一路的印记。

我不知道，或许我永远也不会知道。

为何这个痛苦的旅程选择了我。

但我要谢谢您，我的上帝。

是您与我同在。

经历了这些磨难后，还有一个问题困扰着我：在这场悲剧里，上帝在哪？一年半后，我仍然没有答案。把它写下来是一件棘手的事情，特别是一想到我对上帝愤怒和他会有怎样的反应时。或者这问题并没有答案。

尽管我从来不是一个热心的基督教徒，但在面对上帝时却是我变得最痛苦的时候。现在，写关于上帝的内容也是我感恩他在我无助无望时一直支持我的方式。

我的父母都是基督教徒，所以我从小就耳濡目染了基督教的价值观。这些观念更多是潜移默化的，而不是教诲。父亲从来不会和我说什么基督之爱或是基督与上帝的关系之类，但他却用实际行动证明了他对上帝的爱意。父亲是个热心肠，同时在邻里间口碑甚佳。有段日子，他还照看了邻居家的小孩，并且十分关心他们。在大部分时间，父亲会主动帮邻居们买些东西。他们生病时，父亲也尽其所能地去帮助他们。让我刮目相看的是，父亲不仅帮助教堂社区里的人，也会帮助那些和他有相同信仰的虔诚的教徒。他耐心、善良、大方，也很少发脾气。当我拿着糟糕的成绩单回到家，上面满是老师批改的红色笔迹，父亲会坐下来，看着报告单和分数，平静地签上名，然后只是对我说："下次再接再厉吧。"

尽管父亲用行动在践行着基督之爱，但很奇怪，对于我来说上帝并不存在。可能是父亲与上帝的联系，促使他去履行基督之爱，但对我来说却不是这样。我曾试着去寻找现实中的上帝。父亲不会或是不能够用我这个年龄能听得懂的话来清楚地表达出上帝对他的教诲。回过头来看，我应该去了解更多的关于上帝的我所崇敬的、积极的那一面，还有他值得我们去崇敬和喜爱的理由。《圣经》说亚当和夏娃犯了原罪，因此我需要得到上帝的宽恕，但我想知道他们俩的罪行和我有什么关系。我不知道福音书上写的是什么意思。因此，每周日到教堂做礼拜只是每周的惯例，对我没有任何精神意义，周日做礼拜，有时是充满乐趣的，有时又极其无聊，但绝大部分时间是没意义的。幸运星期五和复活节星期天会被简化成用邦尼兔和彩蛋庆祝。圣诞节只不过是比其他节日多了一点点食物和乐趣罢了。回想小的时候，我发现教堂里的大人们，包括我周日学校的老师们，都没用对我而言有意义的方式向我解释过神。他们没有向我解释过人的原罪，也没有解释过为什么耶稣必须死在十字架上。也许，他们对自己的信仰也不知所以然。即便如此，我还是会乖乖地和父亲继续去教堂做礼拜。

青春期的时候，我不断质疑上帝和宗教。作为一个理想主义和对现实充满焦虑的年轻人，我决定不再去教堂，没有人能够说服我，即便是我的父亲。母亲在我幼时自杀，让我感觉自己与其他朋友们不一样。尽管她的离去对于我而言并不像父亲的离去那样具有灾难性，我还是会嫉妒那些有完整家庭的朋友。家里窘迫的经济条件亦令我自卑。人们参加父亲主持的礼拜时都会顺便捎些零钱来。有些人默默捐款，而有些不是私下给父亲钱，而是不顾及父亲的感受公开捐钱，以彰显他们的慷慨大方。我十分厌恶这些，可父亲没有理由去拒绝那些捐款，所以他只能一脸痛苦沮丧的样子站在那里，特别是那些人把所有零钱都乱七八糟地塞给他时。我认为那些基督教徒言行不一，他们的热心助人更多是出于责任，而不是爱，或者更可能是出于他们需要表现出这么慷慨。如果基督教的本质是爱，那我发誓我绝对没有感受到他的存在。我不想成为基督教徒，也不想成为其中一员。让父亲失望的是，那时的我已决定不再因为必须去而去教堂了，要去也得我心甘情愿地去，但那时我已经不再想去了。

在我青少年期的后面几年里，我都没有去过教堂。回过头来看，其实那"荒诞"的几年对我来说倒挺有必要。远离常规教育和教堂的成规，我开始思考关于上帝的事情和上帝在我生活中的意义，我无法理解自己内心的空虚。我认为，在日常的吃喝玩乐、学习、睡觉和生老病死之外，生活中还应该有更多其他的东西。在我受邀请参加了一场由美国的一位福音传道士传播上帝福音的讲座后，我的想法发生了转变。他讲得简洁、真诚，让人听上去非常投入。我渐渐明白，自己其实和所有人一样，都需要得到上帝的仁慈和怜悯。我第一次明白了福音是什么，在上帝的普天之爱下，我显得多么微不足道啊！我同时意识到我没有权利去批判那些基督教徒的弱点。就在那时我认识了苏，一个比我大一些的女生，后来我们成了朋友。她的行为和表现让我从她身上体会到了上帝的爱。我曾见过几次她和受助者接触，她持之以恒的关怀和无微不至的照顾给我留下了很深的印象。同时，她让我恢复了对基督的信念。苏用我能理解的方式和我谈论了她的信仰。

在离开教堂服务四年后的某个星期天，我重新回到了教堂参与服务。我决定成为一名基督教徒，那一天，牧师给我施礼，那一年，我20岁。这一次是我自己做出的决定。我决定去相信上帝因为我想要这么做，而不是我必须这么做。

我想我做得还不错，因为我定期去教堂，还研究《圣经》。我甚至成了主日学校的老师。由于我的经验不足，所以，我要确保每一个在我课上听讲的孩子都能得到我的关注。我很注意去和每一位孩子聊天，去更好地了解他们。那时我已经结婚，并有了三个孩子。这些事情对我来说都不是问题。生活就像波澜不惊的一面湖水，自然而然，我认为自己的信仰是很坚定的。我过着基督徒的生活，上帝在我的心中，还有什么挑战是我不能克服的呢？

然而父亲的自杀，就是其中一个（我难以克服的挑战①）。父亲的自杀打破了我以往舒适平静的生活。这些年研读《圣经》并没让我有能力来解释这些难题：为什么上帝让这件事情发生在我身上？为什么他不仅带走了母亲，还带走了父亲？这是惩罚吗？这是诅咒吗？父母的自杀让我开始怀疑上帝的爱和他的法力无边。如果他宣称的全能、全知和无处不再是可信的，那为什么他不阻止我父母自杀？他真的是善良的吗？我可以在别人遭遇不幸时引用圣经条文，滔滔不绝地和他谈论关于上帝的陈词滥调。但在父亲自杀后，我却陷入了信仰危机。母亲去世时我只有两个问题：她会去天堂吗？我可以再见到她吗？那些年我问过不同的人这些问题，也很满意他们的回答。但当父亲也因为自杀去世时，我不得不从精神和情感上面对父母双双自杀的事实。

我诅咒上帝。许许多多的问题和思想矛盾折磨了我好几个月。幸运的是，那段时间，蒂娜一直在我身边陪伴着我。她一直耐心地听我的满腹牢骚，不论我表现出来多么不讨人喜欢，她一如既往地爱着我。她的宽容大度，就像是上帝给予我的爱。我们在一起谈论许多关于父亲自杀的事情，关于这件事情对我和整个家庭的影响。我们谈论上帝，谈论我对他的愤怒，还有我对上帝没能阻止悲剧发生的愤慨。蒂娜耐心地听着，从来不为上帝辩护。我猜，她知道上帝不需要别人为他辩护，上帝自有安排。她泰然面对我的沉默、愤怒和泪水，我非常感激她陪伴我度过的时光。我记得，蒂娜很多次在我不断哭泣时递上纸巾。

---

① 译者注

蒂娜的支持是我在精神之旅中重要的转折点，让我重新信仰上帝。但我从怀疑到信任的转变并非一夜之间就实现的。相反地，这是我在认真审视自己处境后所做出的清醒的决定。在困顿于很多没有答案的问题一段时间之后，我最终接受了上帝的旨意。我有限的思考永远也不可能了解神的计划和意图。莫名其妙地，当我开始决定要放手和"遵照神的旨意"时，我开始感到自己没有那么累了。

一天，我开车去一个地方。一想到父亲和他的惨死，我的眼泪就夺眶而出。我好想他。似乎有什么东西在我脑海中闪过，我抬头看着天空，并开始哀悼起父亲来。乌云的边际镶着一道银边。那一刻，我感觉到上帝在和我说些什么。一直以来，我都只关注自己，认为自己是那么的悲惨。而就在那一天，我忽然意识到上帝才是创造万物的主，他当然知道我所承担的痛苦有多少。想到这儿，我内心的痛苦得到了释放，尽管我无法用言语逻辑解释那一刻我所感受到的平静。

有些读者可能觉得难以理解我信仰的转变。这甚至听起来像是陈腔滥调。我只能说，这些都是我的真实体验。我选择去相信上帝，相信他是至高无上的，一切都是他最好的安排，虽然他的安排对我来说看起来很不幸。

直到现在，我都不能理解为什么上帝会让我父母双双自杀。正因如此，我的疗伤之旅才会被疑虑、不坚定的信仰和许多难以回答的问题所困扰。但我坚信，终有一日，一切都将会有圆满的答案。而那一天，也将是这段旅程的终点。有时，上帝只会在那里沉默不语。在父亲死后，有无数个夜晚，我因为恐惧和焦虑缠身，彻夜未眠。我记得我曾经哭着向上帝请求，请求他让我睡着。大多数晚上，当我平静下来的时候，我还是能够睡着的，只是会容易惊醒，然后又迷迷糊糊地入眠，但也有时候我根本睡不着。有时候，尤其当我留出时间来安静地感应上帝时，我的心情平静了下来，我也感应到了上帝的存在。我多次提醒自己，我终究会到达彼岸的，那只不过是时间问题，上帝仍然在关心着我——尽管他沉默——既然我决意相信他，那么我就应当继续和他并肩前行。

我还能从《圣经》的一些章节中得到慰藉。对我特别有用的是哥林多后书第十二章第九段："我的慈悲慷惠与你，我的力量在弱者身上法力全开。"上帝并不允诺我们一生都没有挑战，但他曾说，在我们痛苦和困惑时他能给予我们力量。

还有其他许多《圣经》上的条文亦让我在旅程中受益良多，例如约伯的故事。他历经苦难，对上帝的信念一再动摇；他失去了财产、儿女、健康——他失去了所有的东西！我遭受的苦难远远不及约伯，但是他的故事让我明白了苦难是我生活中的一部分。或许上帝已经通过我父母自杀的事情告诉我这一点了。又或许他是在告诉我要停下脚步，观察人生，看看自己是否本末倒置了。我经常在忙，忙着追逐生活琐事，而忘了什么才是真正重要的东西。父亲去世后，我一直很后悔以前没有多陪陪他。我和他之间的关系比那些鸡毛蒜皮的小事更加重要，这是毋庸置疑的。现在，我就尽可能花时间和我所爱的人们相处。回过头来看，直到失去我生命中那么重要的一个人之后，我才明白要珍惜感情，这是多么可悲啊！

又一次，上帝在我向他哭诉时回到了我的身边。如果我的人生一帆风顺，我就永远不会有和上帝这么近距离接触的机会，甚至可能将他遗忘。我知道，我可能会继续纠结于他的美德是否真实存在。但我同时也知道，某种程度上来说是确切地知道，上帝比我脆弱的信仰和疑惑更加强大。他曾许诺，他会在我无助无望时给予我无限慈悲的力量。

丧亲之痛后，我的另一个积极的改变是在面对其他和我有类似遭遇的人时更有同情心了。曾经的我是一个极为傲慢的人，十分独立，拒绝依赖他人。然而，在我悲痛不已，不得不寻求咨询师和伙伴的帮助时，我才意识到了人文关怀的重要性。这也让我可以更好地去帮助其他曾经遭遇不幸的人。我现在的心态比以前平和多了。以前，我都致力于"给予"（别人帮助[①]）；现在，我也学会了如何"接受"（别人帮助）。上帝一直在帮助我。父亲自杀带给我的悲痛帮助我成长为一个更好的人。

除了《圣经》，在这场信仰危机中，还有其他书伴我成长。我有幸阅读了肖·露西写的《黑暗中的上帝》一书。一位朋友在很久之前读过，他推荐这本书给我，认为它能帮助到我。肖·露西，一个演说家、诗人、作家和编辑。她作为丈夫的护理人，在书中记录了她与她患癌丈夫一起度过

---

① 译者注，下同

的最后时光。露西在书中只是客观记录了她在丈夫化疗期间经历的痛苦和悲伤，而没有就信仰问题给出答案。我发现，在关于上帝的问题上，露西显得十分虔诚。她描述了自己对上帝的怀疑和愤怒，告诉了我个人应该如何处理与上帝的关系。质疑上帝不一定是缺乏信仰，而是不断地坚定信仰。

C.S. 刘易斯，一位哲学家，同时也是科幻小说的作者，主要撰写儿童书籍和有关基督教的读物。他在其中一本著作《伤痛的问题》中写道："上帝在我们喜悦时细语，在我们悲痛时大斥，以唤起理智；这是他在用扩音喇叭唤醒一个已失聪的世界。"我经常听不到或听不清上帝的话语，因为我在选择性地倾听。我真不知道这会带来什么。或许不断地参与施舍活动能够给我带来满足感。我祈祷上帝不要再用扩音喇叭和我讲话了，即使在没有这种扩音喇叭的情况下，我也会对他的声音非常敏感。

阿伦德·丹，是我最喜欢的基督教书的作者之一，他在《治愈之路》中写道："上帝让我们在生命中受到伤害并因此心痛，这一点让我们困惑。可奇怪的是，在我们失去的同时，他用一种神秘而疯狂的方式让我们确信他的爱。疯狂！上帝先扰乱我们的心，继而争取我们的信任，最后取得我们的信任。"

不管遗属们的信仰和背景有何不同，大家所经历的磨难大同小异，在精神层面也是如此。我分享这段精神之旅，并不是说我已经都有了答案。我仍然因为上帝是否良善、他为何让悲剧发生等问题纠结。我知道，只要我还活着，我就会一直受这怀疑论调的影响。我的心境会随着外部因素摇摆不定，但我内心还是选择了去相信上帝永生常存。

在疗愈的挣扎中，有些东西阻止我继续前行。在与奥菲利娅的会谈疗程里，我的愤怒不断被激化。我们探寻愤怒的根本原因，也知道饶恕他人才能拯救自己的这个道理。理论上我同意她的观点。但我却没有行动的勇气和力量。虽然我也想尽快从愤怒的泥淖中挣脱出来，事实上有时我也是这么做的，但我始终认为自己有理由愤怒。我仍然坚信我不能够说服自己去宽恕他人，认为只有后悔自己做错事的人才会有信念和宽恕的愿望。对于我而言，所有做错事的人都会令我感到愤慨。在一次与奥菲利娅特别艰难的辅导咨询后，这个困惑得以解决，那天回到家后，我十分沮丧，我什么都不想做，只想看看书让自己平静下来。这一直是我碰到困难时逃避现实的一种方法。我在想念和父亲相处的故地时，弗雷德里克·比克纳所著的书《家的渴望》① 吸引了我的注意。在比克纳还很小的时候他的父亲自杀了。书中有一个章节"通往圆满的旅程"，阐述了上帝对于可恶的罪人是何等的仁慈。我数月不能理解宽恕的本质，看完这一章节后，我开始理解了。在书中比克纳问道："一个支离破碎的世界怎么可能变得圆满？难道是苦思冥想和痛苦？难道是独身一人的大慈大悲？又难道是人类永远无法到达的境地？"

比克纳引用了卡拉马佐夫兄弟的故事（陀思妥耶夫斯基虚构）。"竹西玛在小说的情节中没有立刻成为一个完整的人。他还有好长的一段路要走，我们亦然。但是上帝的仁慈不但让他看到了如天堂般的世界，更为他的心灵打开了天堂的大门……陀思妥耶夫斯基想告诉我们，通往圆满的旅程就是我们和竹西玛学会去同情他人、爱他人的过程。"

不知道怎么地，那些天我的愤怒都消失了。对我来说，经历这场心的体验和转变真是个奇迹。持续不断的痛苦和愤恨被爱和同情心代替，曾经愤怒的心也温柔了起来。我没有逼迫自己去宽恕；相反地，我是被内心的一股使命所驱动。也许，我看到了自己不可理喻的一面，看到了自己同其他人一样，是多么需要仁慈和宽恕之心。

在父亲葬礼的那一天，蒂娜给了我一封信。这封信给了我安慰，现在看来，这封信更是意味深远。她在信上是这么写的：

亲爱的尹：

今天早上我想到了以下两点：

1. 你的父亲不用再因为身体衰老虚弱而受罪了。他现在是自由的、无拘无束的，他可以尽情跳舞了。

2. 你父亲去世时，爱耶稣之人必然和你感同身受。对于他们来说，简直就是世界末日一般。他们看到的只有黑暗和绝望。你父亲死得这么悲惨，他们必然也同样为此感到悲痛。

---

① 原文 A Longing For Home，应为 The Longing For Home，

但死亡并不是故事的终点。他的死亡我们已经无法掌控，而爱仍然让我们为他的离去而痛苦万分。

所以，尽管泪水朦胧了我们的双眼，悲伤和痛苦蒙蔽了我们的心灵，但你父亲的故事绝不会就此画上句号。他的一生，还有你们（不仅是他的孩子们，还包括他的女婿和儿媳们，以及他的孙子和外孙们）对他的爱，都是他生命的见证。在你母亲离开后，你父亲克服艰难险阻，在极度困难的经济条件下，含辛茹苦地将你们抚养长大。他养育了爱主的第二代，现在第二代又开始养育第三代。

我们都深深感受到了你的丧父之痛。他是一名慈爱的父亲，失去他是多么令人痛心疾首。痊愈需要时间。也许那些伤痛会一直存在，但绝不会一直这么的疼。

上帝并没有抛弃你。你的父亲并没有抛弃你。他的离去给你带来了巨大的伤害。但我想，他内心是为了你好。

我和所有爱你的人与你同在。

蒂娜

第六章
时间如何平复一切？

一年过去了，新的一年又来临，
然而对于我来说却都一样。
我痛过、哭过，
我努力地搜寻，
期待奇迹的出现，
哪怕只是一点点机会，
我想再见到那个身影，
哪怕是匆匆一瞥，
对我来说，却已弥足珍贵。

哪里才没有他的身影呢？
我走进每一间房子，到处都有他的记忆。
多么痛苦的渴望啊！
我的心在收缩，
我看不见他，无论我如何凝视。
我感觉他就在我的身后，
我听见他爬楼梯的声音，
这个房子里都是他的一颦一笑，
但他再也不在了。

在回忆中生活

时间不知不觉地流逝，一天、一周、一个月，然后到了父亲的一周年、两周年忌日。我没有哪一天不想念父亲。我的记忆停留在他活着的时候；停留在病痛使他忧郁与绝望的时候；停留在他因挫败而流泪、害怕和伤心的时候；停留在他结束自己生命的那一天。我一度怀疑这些记忆会伴随很长一段时间。时间的确能疗伤，但永远抹不掉我对父亲的爱与他自杀带给我的伤痛。

我觉得很神奇，没有父亲的安慰陪伴我居然可以活下去。若是没有朋友们、其他遗属们和新加坡援人协会的心理咨询师的支持与肯定，我可能仍然还困在父亲自杀的阴影中。在父亲去了天堂两年后，我写了这本书，我仍然在想念他。但逐渐地，我更多地追忆和父亲在一起时的幸福时光。我偶尔会强烈地感觉到他已不在我身边，会因此感到痛苦，有时我甚至会哭。但这些悲伤再也压不垮我，我记住了他的音容笑貌，父亲永远活在我的心中。

就像爬螺旋楼梯一样，我会继续重温这些感觉，但每一次都会从不一样的更高视野的层面去看。当父亲健在时，每周他会在我家待上一天。在他刚去世后的几个月里，一想到他再也不会出现在我家了，我就难以忍受，所以我每次都会把这些想法抛得远远的。我不愿想起他每周在我家的日子，因为他的离去使我太悲痛了。然而现在我会想起和珍藏他在我家时的记忆。那时，我们也没做什么特别的事，就是整天做些寻常的事情：父亲看他最喜欢的电视节目，有时下厨做做饭。他在我家很随意，会在房间和花园里四处走走，有时候会在我忙于家务时帮我打理一下花园。

在国外度假时发生了与记忆中相同的事。在父亲离开大约一年后，我觉得我需要来一场旅行。我以为离开一段时间我会暂时忘记父亲自杀的事情，从沉痛的悲伤中走出来一会儿。然而结果却是，在旅途中，我又回想起跟父亲一起到国外度假的情景。我很伤心，因为再也不能同父亲旅游了。一路上风景变幻多端，按理来说多少能分散些我的注意力，让我不再总去回忆失去父亲的痛苦，丈夫和孩子们也很努力地想让我旅程过得开心，而我却依旧沉溺在对父亲的回忆里。我想起出行前帮他收拾行李。他总是轻装上阵但会小心翼翼地带上足够的御寒衣服，因为他怕冷。我记得那时我们拿东西特别慢，因为父亲那个时候动作非常缓慢，还固执得拒绝使用轮椅或拐杖。父亲年纪大，飞机的经济舱座位坐着很不舒服，但他从不抱怨,飞机餐提供什么他就吃什么,尽管他平时挺挑食。到达目的地后,由于寒冷的天气他情愿待在室内,但在我们的鼓励下他也会勇敢地跟我们一同外出。我会帮他穿得暖暖的,让他不会感到寒冷。他会无微不至地帮朋友跟家人选购礼物!旅途中,这些往事的点点滴滴激发了我强烈的悲伤与失落感。这个假期对我来说并不开心。

但一年后,我的全家第二次旅行时,感觉却很不同。由于我丈夫工作的原因,我们去了美国并在那里住了几年。我想起父亲去看望我们的情形,想起他怎么适应新环境、食物、寒冷天气和人。我清楚地记得父亲开怀大笑、微笑着享受与家人在一起的时光。最重要的是,我清楚地记得父亲与朋友和国外的亲戚谈论起自己家庭时脸上流露出的满足与自豪。

节点

虽然对于遗属来说,重拾生活的勇气是一个很大的挑战,但我发现,在疗愈悲伤的路上总会遇到各种节点。我接受辅导,希望能尽快结束悲伤的旅程,希望到了父亲的一周年忌日时自己可以好起来。我甚至还觉得若是我能通过第一年这个坎我就会变好,我的生活将会回归正常的轨道。这是我为自己设立的节点。结果必然是一个错误的预判。通过我自己和其他遗属的经历,我现在才知道这些节点并非以时间来划分。一些遗属可能会比其他人更快地迈过生命中的这道坎,而且每个遗属的节点都不同,但仍然有些遗属的节点与我相似。

挠人的回忆消失了

我疗愈旅程中的一个节点是那些挠人的回忆消失了。在悲伤初期,我不断地想起我最后见到父亲健在的那一天。我不断地在脑海里想起他,想起那天早上我是如何帮他从床上坐起来,因为他再也没力气自己坐起来了,还想起他在我离开时怎样说再见。那幅画面和那一声"好的"不断地在我脑海里回放。我控制不住一遍又一遍地回放,但有一天,这些挠人的回忆突然不再出现了。我不记得是什么时候开始的,但我知道那些天当我想重温过去的这些回忆时，我却不得不刻意地去回想当时的情景：它们再也没有闪现在我的脑海里了。我有时也会再唤醒这些回忆，因为我不想失去跟父亲最后一天相处的记忆。我偶尔还会唤醒这些记忆来使我的心变得柔软一些——提醒我要更加同情和理解那些刚蒙受痛苦的遗属。

我也注意到，跟父亲最后一天相处的记忆不再像之前那么让我痛苦。一开始的时候，每每回忆起来，我就会有很多消极的想法，特别悔恨内疚。但现在这些消极的思想已经大大减少并且我几乎不觉得内疚了。在父亲自杀两年后，我可以坦然地说我那时已经竭尽所能了。

我也会回想并且沉浸在美好的回忆中——我们一起外出，一起出国旅游，一起在他的公司看电视，开车载上父亲一起外出。在父亲刚走的几个月内，只要我试图回忆那些美好的日子，我都会陷入一种"要是……就好了"的混乱境地，并且跌落到痛苦的回忆当中。

一开始，我每周都要去父亲的墓前看看，以这种方式来跟他保持联系。他的一周年忌日后，我已经能够减少去看望他的次数，只在一些重要的日子才会去。我不必为了跟父亲保持联系而待在那里。当我需要想念他时，他就活在我的心中与脑海里。

托尼，一个父亲自杀的遗属，在回忆方面跟我有着惊人的相似之处。在他父亲跳楼后的几个月里，当他收到坏消息时他的脑海里不断地想起他们最后一刻的对话。他发现跟心理咨询师面谈几次后，他开始能够阻止自己想起那些父亲自杀的画面了。当那些挠人的回忆消失时，他可以更好地思考和管理自己的悲伤情绪。他也不再每天都去父亲的墓碑前停留了。

触景伤情少了

王太太谈起她以前是如何努力回避那些让她想起儿子的人。她避开她的侄子，避开那些孩子与她儿子同龄的朋友。但三年后，她甚至能与他们同处一室并互相打招呼，尽管她还做不到与他们交谈。

在有些地方见到有些人，会让遗属触景伤情，这一点我也经历过。一开始的时候我几乎不敢见我的兄弟们，因为我害怕一见到他们，就会想起父亲自杀后，我们在父亲的公寓里、在父亲的灵堂和葬礼上待在一起的痛苦回忆。大概一年半以后，在家庭聚会上再见到他们时我便不那么害怕了。尽管我们还是回避父亲自杀的话题，但我已经不必再躲开他们了。

有时候，某些事情已不再刺激到我。这几天走过父亲常去的理发店时，想到他已离去，我也不再那么痛苦。我可能会突然想起他，但这些念头会一闪而过，我可以继续做原本要做的事。我也会去以前经常光顾的鱼贩子那里买鱼，看到他已不再让我伤感，虽然这些天没有父亲的陪伴我几乎不买他的鱼。

一起伸出援手

在疗愈旅程中，我们当中的一些人已经达到了一种认识的高度，我们没有被悲伤所淹没，同时我们还帮助其他人。那些悲剧让我们比别的不幸的人更加敏感，并且深深地渴望去帮助别人。王太太跟大家谈起她在工作中接触到一个完全陌生的人，他母亲因病去世了，他觉得王太太的帮助让他很感动，并在她的老板面前称赞她。希拉开始去倾听和安慰被病魔夺去母亲的邻居，她怀疑如果不是因为她自己经历过类似的痛苦，她根本无法做得这么好。阿莲和乔安妮自愿成为"疗愈桥"小组的辅导员，并且她们也愿意让那些遗属在除了"疗愈桥"之外的其他私人时间找她们。她们在分享环节仍然会哭，但是她们已经变得足够强大，可以去安慰那些新加入的遗属。

悲伤的往事过去一年半后，奥菲利娅让我和她一起去当"疗愈桥"小组的辅导员。我非常愿意，因为我相信在互助会中我能发挥出作用。这对我来说是一个很重要的转折点，因为我终于能够在悲痛的同时和其他遗属们一起努力。

2007 年，我人生第一次公开谈论我的不幸。新加坡援人协会专门为自杀者的遗属们组织了一个论坛，为了让他们听听老遗属的经历。我同意作为四个分享经验的"疗愈桥"小组成员之一，同他们分享我们的故事，并且回答他们提出的我们是如何应对痛苦的问题。我们也想让新成员知道他们在悲痛中并不孤单，他们可以在这里得到支持。在我的疗愈旅程中，相信自己并不孤单对我的治疗起了很关键的作用，正因为如此，我决定不去过多介意自己的隐私，与他们分享，只要这能帮助到他们。自杀的悲剧同样也会发生在他们的身上——好父亲、好母亲、好孩子们以及所爱之人自杀的人们。当我在二十多位参加论坛的新遗属面前分享自己的故事时，我哭了。同时，我很高兴能帮助他们理解并邀请他们参加互助会。

这不是结束

成为自杀者遗属的经历就像是一场违背了我意愿的旅行。在旅行刚开始的时候，我设定了个目标，希望一切变得美好，过去的就让它抛诸脑后，当这些遭遇结束，我还能够继续过着阳光和幸福的生活。但之后我才意识到，前路漫漫，这是一生的旅途。

海伦·凯勒，一个非凡的美国妇女，一出生就是聋哑人，但她在逆境中拼搏，学会了说话、阅读、写字。她说："我们已经享受过的是不会失去的。我们深爱的一切已经成为我们的一部分。"我是在新加坡援人协会的小册子上第一次看到这句话。一想到即使父亲不在了，但他的价值观和他所代表的一切，将永远活在我的记忆与生活里，我的心满是慰藉。

从这个意义上来讲，在真正意义上，父亲永远活着我心中！

致　谢

致我的丈夫和孩子，当我整天魂不守舍的时候，谢谢你们对我的爱、理解和鼓励。

致蒂娜，我最亲爱的朋友，谢谢你从开始到现在一直陪伴着我。没有你的友谊、耐心和爱，这次的人生旅程不知将要把我带至何方。

致奥菲利娅，我的新加坡援人协会的咨询师，你的毅力和耐心总让我震惊。谢谢你相信我、指导我并给我信心去完成这本书，并在此过程中让我在遭受父母双双自杀的痛苦后，还相信一切都会好起来。

致同为遗属的兄弟姐妹们，谢谢你们与我一路同行。你们活下去的勇气还有助人的愿望深深地激励着我。

致上帝，尽管到现在，我依然不清楚您为什么会让这样的悲剧发生，但我感谢您在我最痛苦和焦虑的时候给了我平静。

关于作者

当尹还只有 7 岁的时候，她的母亲自杀了。而四十年后，她的父亲也跳楼自杀。本书所讲的就是她如何从双亲自杀而亡的阴影中走出来的故事。当时尹 47 岁，在成为家庭主妇前，她曾是一名理疗师。她结婚了，有了三个孩子，他们分别是 20 岁、18 岁和 16 岁。

翻译词汇对照表

Samaritans Of Singapore（SOS）　新加坡援人协会（简称SOS）

Yin　尹

Cantonment Close　广东民弄

early onset of dementia　早期痴呆症

Survivor　遗属

Insomnia　失眠症

Paranoia　妄想狂；偏执狂

Changi　（新加坡）樟宜

East Coast　（新加坡）东海岸

the Healing Bridge　康复桥

Tina　蒂娜

Mary Mathew　玛丽·马修

Ophelia　奥菲利娅

Elizabeth Kubler Ross　伊丽莎白·库伯·罗斯

On Death and Dying　《论生死和临终》

Healing Bridge　疗愈桥

Sheila　希拉

Joanne　乔安妮

Jascintha　雅辛塔

Gan　阿甘

Joseph	约瑟夫
Nick	尼克
Choo	周
Lian	阿莲
Sue	苏
The Bible	圣经
Adam and Eve	亚当和夏娃
Christian	耶稣
2nd Corinthians	哥林多后书
Job	约伯
Luci Shaw	肖·露西
God In The Dark	《黑暗中的上帝》
C. S. Lewis	C. S. 刘易斯
The Problem Of Pain	《伤痛的问题》
Dan Allender	阿伦德·丹
The Healing Path	《治愈之路》
A Longing For Home	《家的渴望》
Frederick Buechner	弗雷德里克·比克纳
The Journey Toward Wholeness	通往圆满的旅程
The Brother Karamazov	卡拉马佐夫兄弟
Dostoyevsky	陀思妥耶夫斯基
Zossima	竹西玛
Helen Keller	海伦·凯勒

WHY?

When Both My Parents Took Their Lives

Yin

This book is lovingly dedicated to the memory of:

My Dad and Mum. Though not with me in person anymore, they live on in my heart and in my memory.

The late Mary Mathew, Executive Director of the Samaritans of Singapore. Her warmth and gentleness as she listened gave me hope that I could survive the ordeal of my parents'suicides.

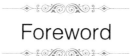

Foreword

When someone dear to us dies through suicide, we are left with the agonising ordeal of having to survive the heart rending loss. It traumatises us and leaves us with a profound struggle to make sense of the suicide and learn to live again.

"Suicide survivors" are those who have been left behind after a suicide and their loss and grief tend to be misunderstood and, sometimes, inappropriately responded to by people who seek to offer comfort and support. There are those who want to help but instead of helping, they could be adding salt to injury, amplifying the pain and grief of suicide survivors.

It is also a struggle for suicide survivors themselves to acknowledge, appreciate and adapt to life after the suicide. Many tend to cope in silence and solitude, left with a sense of bewilderment as to what had happened.

Perhaps what is needed is to give voice to those who are suicide survivors and hear their arduous journey towards healing. This is Yin's attempt in offering us the opportunity to journey with her as she shares her story and that of others like her.

I count it a privilege to be associated with Samaritans of Singapore and be offered the opportunity of experiencing this journey through Yin's account of her healing process. Her candid disclosure of her struggles is most engaging, inviting me and you into the inner world of her experience in healing from the trauma as a survivor of her father's suicide.

This first-hand narration of Yin promises not only to enlighten, but also serves as a balm for those working through their own loss and grief.

I am grateful for Yin's contribution to SOS, and for the work of all others who offer a healing hand to those left behind in the aftermath of suicide.

May you journey with Yin and others like her by sharing this book with fellow sojourners who may be experiencing loss and grief.

Anthony Yeo

Chairman and Consultant,

Samaritans of Singapore

Consultant Therapist,

Counselling and Care Centre

Preface

My dad's suicide overwhelmed me with sadness, grief, and regrets. I was on an emotional roller coaster and felt extremely lost. A friend suggested that I talk to a counsellor from the Samaritans of Singapore (SOS). After much resistance and hesitation, I called the SOS and soon found myself embarking on a journey that was painful and tiring, but necessary for my healing.

The idea of writing this book was mooted by Ophelia, my SOS counsellor. At first I was reluctant. It was different from the simpler process of keeping a journal, in which I just scribbled whatever came to my mind or my heart——whatever overwhelmed me. It had been difficult enough coping with the memories that kept replaying in my mind. Writing a book about my dad's suicide meant summoning these painful memories and walking repeatedly through the whole nightmare. The thought of sitting down, recalling and recording the memories was frightening. The fear was apparent in my procrastination. I told myself that it was too painful to write about Dad's suicide, that I was not a writer, and that I was too ambitious to even consider writing a book. I had never undertaken a project of this magnitude. But a part of me realised that this was perhaps one way of making something useful out of the tsunami that had swept through my life, and that it would be of some comfort to other survivors who felt alone in their experience of suicide grief.

At first, I could not even bring myself to write the word "suicide". Each time I used that word, Dad's death rushed to the forefront and blocked out everything else. My grief engulfed me, and I could not focus on the writing process. I resorted to using the letter "s" as a substitute, until it became more bearable to see the word on the computer screen.

There were times when I thought of aborting this project altogether, because the writing took me to deep and sad places. But looking back, I am glad I persevered because the writing became increasingly therapeutic. It provided an additional outlet for my thoughts and feelings. I could take my time, write when I felt like it and stop when I needed a break. Sure, there were tears. But there were also good memories such as his fatherly gentleness when he took me out for special treats, just the two of us, father and child. Those were special times when I felt singled out and especially loved.

Writing this book also became a journey during which I explored undiscovered areas of my life. I must add that I am not proud of some of these discoveries, but I now know myself better and I have learnt to like myself more.

So this book is my gift to myself and other survivors.

Yin September 2008

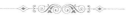

Contents

Chapter 1

Why, Dad?

We met in a room in the Samaritans of Singapore (SOS) office in Cantonment Close. Prying eyes were kept out by curtains. Some drinks and several boxes of tissues were on the table before us. We were there to share our painful stories. I had hoped that my presence would be a source of some comfort to the other survivors. I could empathise with my fellow survivors as they spoke of their pain, helplessness, emptiness and emotional upheaval because I had been there. As I listened to their stories, it became clear to me that the support of fellow survivors was very crucial in such a daunting and lonely a journey. But my being there also hurled me back to that fateful day when I became a survivor. The day of my Dad's suicide was the start of a lonely journey with an unknown destination.

Before that day

My Dad had not been well for almost two years before his death. He was in his late 80s, and with every weekly visit, I noticed a decline in his general health. He was in constant pain and discomfort in the weeks leading to his suicide. He was physically weak, emotionally and mentally fragile, and spiritually challenged. To my Dad, his prayers were not answered and he became increasingly discouraged and frustrated with his condition. He was fearful of the future.

The geriatrician's diagnosis was depression with an early onset of dementia. The visits to the doctors did little to ease his complaints about his ailments. Seeing his progressive deterioration to only a shadow of his former self saddened me beyond words. On the numerous occasions when we talked, Dad frequently expressed a deep desire for God to take him to his heavenly home. He was tired of living.

Deep within my heart, I knew that he missed my Mum very much. He had been a widower for many years and had been lonely for a long time. He used to reminisce about Mum. Theirs was an arranged marriage. He had agreed to marry her without seeing her in person. She was several years his junior, pretty, and had completed High School in China. When Mum died, she was cremated, and her ashes was placed in a columbarium. Dad reserved a niche next to hers and he looked forward to taking his place there if only God would take him. But God did not grant him what he most desired. Neither did God answer my prayer to ease Dad into eternity without suffering. I had thought it was merely a question of time before God heard us. What I did not know was that secretly, Dad had decided to hasten his transition from this world to the next, so that he could be with God, so that he could be with Mum.

Dad and I were very close and I could never imagine life without him, even though at the back of my mind, I knew that he was advanced in years and poor in health. When I lost my Mum at the age of seven, he became both father and mother to me. He cooked and saw me off to school. In my turbulent adolescent years, he was unwavering in his fatherly love. He was my confidante in my childhood years and I in turn was his confidante in the autumn of his life. When he passed away, not by sickness or by old age, but because he chose to take his own life, it shattered my world.

That day

The fateful day started out like an ordinary weekday with routine chores. After sending my children to school, I went to the wet market to buy fresh food for Dad's maid to cook for him. When I arrived at his apartment, Dad was still lying in bed; lately he had been spending an inordinate amount of time in bed. Sleep eluded him night and day. He was extremely agitated. We spent some time talking and I tried to lift his spirits. But inside me, I felt helpless as ever, because I knew he was going through a very difficult time and there was little I could do to comfort him. Dad had always treasured his independence, but he had now reached a stage where he had to rely on others to help him perform even basic personal tasks. This affected his self-esteem. He became despondent.

Because of his insomnia, Dad could not get adequate rest. Paranoia set in. He was suspicious of the people around him, and he was unhappy with practically everything. I sensed that his life was devoid of meaning for him, that it had become increasingly unbearable to go on living. I had a difficult time adjusting to the change in his behaviour. Dad used to be logical, compassionate, kind, gentle, godly, prayerful, and much more. I grieved the loss of my Dad at this point of his life. Even though he was physically present, he was not the Dad that I knew. But I realised that was the time he most needed my care and understanding. So I had this quiet resolve in my heart to do my best for him by making his remaining days as bearable and comfortable as possible.

That day, like so many days before, I sat on Dad's bed. I spoke to him and tried to interest him in bits of daily news. I patted him to sleep. Our roles had reversed: I was like a parent to him and he the child. How I wish I could recapture the times when he was his old hearty self.

Despite my efforts to soothe him and induce sleep, he was very restless. He told me that he had no appetite and was always feeling very tired. I fed him some essence of chicken, hoping that it would strengthen him, at least for the day. As I had to attend to other errands, I told him that I had to go and that I would see him again another day. He seemed his usual self as he bade me goodbye. That was the last time I fed my dad, the last time I touched him, the last time I heard his voice, and the last time I saw him alive. The image and memory of that last contact has never left me-we had said our last goodbye.

Several hours later, when I was on another errand, I received a phone call from my elder brother. He lived with Dad, so a call from him would usually be an update about Dad and his condition. Sometimes, he just needed to vent his frustrations and helplessness as a primary caregiver. So I was prepared to hear him out on my earpiece as I continued driving.

"Dad has jumped down," he said. I could not believe what I was hearing.

"What do you mean he has jumped down?" The news hit me so hard that I had to stop driving and pulled to the side of the road. My heart was racing and I was paralysed with fear. I remember screaming and crying into the phone and asking him question after question: "Why? How could this have happened? Where was the maid? Why didn't she stop him?"

The image that immediately flashed through my mind was that of Dad during his last moments just before he jumped. How did he drag himself to the window? He was physically very weak when I left him that morning. He barely had the energy to sit up in bed. How did he climb up the window ledge? He must have harnessed every remaining bit of his strength to manage that last physical task. In my mind I kept seeing him jump, again and again. I could not shake off that horrid image. Question after question raced through my mind. Why did this happen? Why did he resort to suicide? Why didn't I see this coming? Why did he give up? Why didn't he tell me? Why did he have to die this way? Oh, how he must have suffered! I was certain that he would not have chosen this tragic way if he had not been terribly desperate and tormented. The thought of my dad struggling with such overwhelming emotional pain amplified the indescribable pain I felt.

From the car, I called my husband at his office; he rushed to my side and together, we drove to Dad's apartment. Wave after wave of intense feelings of guilt, regret and an utter sense of loss and hopelessness hit me as we made our way there. At the same time, I could not believe that this had actually happened.

When we arrived, I couldn't bring myself to see his body. How could it be that he was alive in the morning but was now gone forever? The fact was cold, cruel, and simply beyond my ability to comprehend emotionally, mentally, and physically. Part of me wanted to see him, to touch him, to be with him. But another part of me wanted to pull away. I did not want to confirm it; I could not bear to confront it. I desperately wanted to continue believing that he was still alive. I was also very afraid of what I might see. Would I still recognise him? Would his body be mangled and bloodied? Would I see bits of him everywhere?

I had contacted my close friend, Tina, who rushed over. Given my state of confusion and fear, I asked whether I should view Dad's body. She was against the idea. She was afraid that I might not be able to cope with what I might see. She asked me to consider whether it would be better for me to remember my Dad as he had been earlier, rather than what he might look like lying on the grass. Today, I'm glad I heeded her advice because I now retain the image of Dad when he was alive, well and whole.

The police were there to conduct their investigation. They were in the apartment and were gathering around the window where Dad had jumped. A stool was next to the window and near the stool, my Dad's slipper; he had left one slipper behind as he clambered up the window ledge. I watched their deliberations from a distance. It was as if I was watching a movie and I was not really there. I was physically there and yet I felt as if I was far away and somehow uninvolved except for those instances when someone spoke to me directly. Even then, I felt as if my clone was answering for me.

The police, of course, had their job to do, but their presence was nevertheless an intrusion to a family in grief. They asked questions in a detached and professional way. Most of their questions were directed at the maid, who was the last person to have seen Dad alive. When the investigation was over, they left after giving us instructions on the procedure for claiming Dad's body from the mortuary the following day.

Every suicide is a police case. An autopsy usually has to be done to exclude foul play. The thought of his frail body being cut open was unthinkable. It did not help that I had heard horrid stories of how autopsies were conducted, and these thoughts assaulted my already battered emotions. Dad had always been a prim and proper person when he was alive and now, there would be strangers looking at his uncovered body, dissecting him. Would they treat his body with the respect he deserved? I felt extremely helpless about the autopsy; there was nothing I could do to protect him; I had no control over this. Irrational as it may seem, I thought of how cold he would be in the morgue with nothing on and no one to keep him warm. Dad, when he was alive, had not liked being in places that were too cold for him. The morgue was a very cold place.

My brothers gave me the task of choosing the clothes that Dad would wear for the last time; I was the youngest of the three siblings, the only girl, and the closest to Dad. I was reluctant and felt extremely sad to have to do it. It was surreal. He was alive this morning, and yet here I was, deciding what he should wear in his casket. How did it come to this? It was difficult to make sense of what was happening.

How do I handle the pain? How could I carry on living knowing that Dad's death by suicide would cast a shadow that would stay with me forever? How could I cope with life, knowing that I would never again be joyful? What would a meaningless existence be like? How could I live with the thought that Dad's suffering had driven him to suicide? There was a fleeting moment when I thought that the only way to escape my pain was to go the same way as Dad, take the plunge and escape the pain I knew I would have to face.

I went home that night feeling extremely tired; my whole being had been assaulted emotionally, mentally and spiritually. I tried to rest, but I drifted between wakeful restlessness and nightmarish sleep.

The following day

When I woke up the following morning, I felt numb and devoid of any feelings. I remember going to the hairdresser to have my hair washed as if nothing had happened. My conversations with the hairdresser were normal and no different from all the previous conversations I had with her. The hairdresser did not detect any trace of sadness and weariness. As on previous occasions, she asked after my Dad's health and as on previous occasions, I replied that he was getting old and frail.

After getting my hair done, I even went grocery shopping. I walked up and down the aisles picking up the usual household items, all the while feeling strangely detached. I was going about my routine as if everything was fine and normal. I even made a phone call to a friend of mine to request that she keep Dad's death to herself and not inform my wider circle of friends because I wanted Dad to have a quiet funeral. I was calm and collected during the telephone conversation. It was as if someone else, not me, was saying all that was needed to be said. I wasn't really there.

Throughout the day, there were numerous calls from my siblings asking for my opinion regarding the funeral arrangements and obituary placements. In some unexplained way, I was able to take the calls with detached composure. I know now that the numbness was part of denial and it was the body's way of preserving my sanity. I remember moving between reality and surrealism and at the same time coping with many other intense feelings. It was exhausting as I vacillated between the real and surreal worlds, trying to make sense of all that was happening. I knew that Dad had died of suicide and yet, at that point, the full impact of his suicide did not hit me at the emotional level. While I could go about doing what I had to do, somewhere at the subconscious level I knew that a tragedy had happened, but I had difficulties coming to terms with it. So, when I was alone or with people who did not know Dad or his death, I was able to function almost normally.

However, reality hit home hard later that afternoon when I was told to be present to receive the casket. At that point, I could not deny the reality anymore. The image of Dad lying still and dead in a casket shattered the other world in which he was still old, frail, but alive. Part of me had somehow been clinging on to the hope this was all a nightmare and that I would wake up and everything would be back to normal again. But to my great distress, it was not a nightmare and there was no more hope.

The family was instructed to be at the place where the wake was to be held. It was to be the first time that we would see Dad in the casket. I felt a heavy sense of dread. I was fearful and a large part of me did not want to be there. I love Dad dearly, and to have to see his lifeless form in the casket was simply too horrifying to contemplate. There was not only fear but confusion as well. I did not want to face the reality of the loss. When I finally saw him lying there, I burst into tears — tears of intense sorrow, regrets and remorse. There was a heavy pain in my chest. My husband hugged and held me tightly to stop me from going under. It was unbelievably difficult to come to terms with the thought that I would never be able to communicate with and care for Dad again. There was no escaping the fact that he would never be alive again; that I would never see or talk to him again. He was in the casket. He was dead.

In the process of making plans for the wake and funeral, my siblings and I were at a loss as to what we should tell our friends and relatives. We were afraid of being judged. How should we respond when asked? Would we be judged as being unfilial and uncaring to the extent that Dad had to resort to suicide because we, his children, did not do our best for him? I was fearful that many uninformed people would draw unfair conclusions. At that time, I did not want to and I did not have the energy to grapple with such questions. Collectively, we agreed to keep Dad's suicide private; we decided that there was no need to tell everyone about it.

Whilst preparing for the wake and trying to make sense of all that had happened, a relative, who somehow knew about the suicide, called me on my mobile phone. Instead of comforting me, she started accusing me of not taking care of Dad. She blamed me for his suicide. I was stunned, bewildered and felt totally sick. The pain she had inflicted was more than I could bear. I felt like someone had dealt a blow to my heart and a deep wave of guilt and sorrow washed over me. Her response reinforced and confirmed the fear I had that survivors would be judged, whether overtly or covertly. It made me more resolved to keep the nature of Dad's death to myself.

The wake

At the wake, I stayed very close to Dad's casket. I wanted to spend whatever remaining time I had with him while he was still physically present. Seeing his lifeless form in the casket evoked intense and painful memories that were beyond words. There was such profound sorrow at a level that I had never ever experienced before.

Each night after the wake service, when friends had dispersed, I would return home feeling emotionally raw and physically drained. I was functioning like a zombie. I could not eat and I barely slept. The little food I ate was forced upon me by my family members. I lost weight but my health was the last thing on my mind.

Two days after Dad's death and after I had returned home from another wake service, the flood-gates opened. I cried non-stop for more than three hours, an unbearable heart-wrenching weeping that came from a sorrow deep inside me. My husband sat with me and held me. The memory of that night, when I mourned the death of my Dad through suicide, still brings tears to my eyes. It was early morning before the tears dried up. There were no tears left and no sleep possible, just a persistent pounding headache.

Friends and relatives who turned up at the wake wanted to know how Dad had died. Their questions put me in a dilemma. Although the family had decided not to mention suicide, a part of me felt that it was not right to lie about his death; yet it was impossible to tell them the truth. So I remained silent whenever the question was asked because I could not make an appropriate response.

The final farewell

The funeral was especially poignant and painful. Dad's pastor comforted us by reminding us that death was not the end of life; he spoke of Dad being in heaven, a place far better than earth. No more sleepless nights for him, no more tears and no more fears. He had been freed from his pain and was no longer bound in his earthly body of weakness and sorrow. He was basking in the presence of God and one day we would meet again.

It was cold comfort; yet I needed to hear it. I needed the assurance that he was in a safe place and that I would one day see him again. It gave me something to hold on to, a place of calm in the rough days ahead. But it did nothing to assuage the sorrow I felt during the funeral service. Physical death was final and nothing could ever reverse that. The whole funeral service signaled the physical separation that would henceforth exist between Dad and myself.

I managed to maintain my composure throughout the service although my tears flowed unceasingly as I thought about Dad's life; how hard he had worked as a single parent to provide for the family.

I knew that I would miss him and the times we had together.

As the casket made its way to the crematorium, I recalled the many trips I had taken with Dad, in Singapore and abroad. I was saddened by the thought that this was his last journey on earth; that he had died alone, without the presence of his loved ones, without me there. I also knew that the journey ahead for me would be difficult and arduous. There was no other way.

Chapter 2

When Love Hurts

Dad's belongings

There seemed to be no end to the crushing reminders that Dad had died through suicide. One depressing reminder came a couple of days after the funeral when the family proceeded to Dad's apartment to sort out his belongings.

His room looked exactly as it had been when he was alive. Nothing in the room had changed except that he was no longer there, and would never be there again. I sat on his bed and held his pillow. I tried hard to summon the memories of my last days with him, to remember what it was like, what he had looked like. I did not want to forget, I was afraid of forgetting, and yet when the memories came flooding back I found them agonising.

Every item of his personal belongings was a brutal reminder that he was gone forever, that he would not be coming back any more. The cup that he had used for many years still bore the stains of his favourite drink. His clothes, which included his Sunday best for going to church, were neatly hung in his cupboard. As I cleared out his cupboard, it struck me that Dad had been a very tidy man. Every item of his clothing was neatly hung. I cried when I saw a sweater that I had bought for him years ago. It was his favourite because it had kept him warm especially in his later years.

He had spent a lot of time in this room when his health deteriorated, when he got weaker and weaker. This was a place where he spent his days and nights, and yet, it was not a peaceful place for him; it was not a place of rest because, tired as he was, sleep eluded him for days on end. This was where he had his meals when he became too weak to even walk the short distance to the dining room. This was where he did his toilet because he was simply too tired to make the trip to the bathroom. How then did he manage to get to the window in the living room all by himself? How did he manage to climb onto the ledge?

His wheelchair, a contraption that he had great disdain for, now sat in a corner of his room, untouched. All attempts to put him in the wheelchair to facilitate his mobility were met with protest. The wheelchair had quickly become a symbol of his declining health and his loss of independence. It was a blow to his self-esteem, and on the rare occasions when he agreed to use it, he did so grudgingly. He preferred to remain immobile indoors than to be taken out in his wheelchair.

As I looked around the room, I saw Dad's old and trusty television set. There was a time when he had been well enough and interested enough to prop himself up on his bed to watch his favourite programmes. However as insomnia and paranoia set in, he lost interest in everything including his regular Tv dramas. Like the wheelchair, the television became a redundant piece of furniture, and now another reminder that he was no longer around to use it.

My eyes rested on Dad's calendar. It was the old-fashioned tear-away calendar with a huge date on each page. Even in his last days, Dad was particular about keeping his calendar current. A page was faithfully torn away every day until the day he died. And that was the last date showing on the calendar. It was as if time had stopped the day he jumped.

reluctantly I went through his personal belongings—the photographs, souvenirs and other knick-knacks that he had accumulated over the years. There were photographs of him when he was a young man. He had cut quite a dashing figure in his youth and I stared long and hard at the person in the photograph, a part of me willing him to come back to life somehow. At that moment, all I wanted was for him to come back so that we could have our usual conversations; I wanted to hear him talk again and tell his stories even if they had become repetitive. I wouldn't mind; I just wanted him back; I would do anything to have him alive again. The pain of my loss and longing was intensified by the inescapable realisation that he had taken his own life. He had committed suicide. These words were a constant refrain in my mind. I desperately needed a second chance to re-write the way his life ended. His life should have and could have ended differently. I sat there, helplessly aware of my inability to change anything that had happened.

It was my job to sift through his belongings and decide what to keep and what to discard. I found that I could not bear the thought of throwing anything away. Getting rid of his possessions would be like wiping out his existence. This was all that was left of Dad and I wanted to hold on to everything to maintain his presence in my life a bit longer. Every item had become more precious by the absence of the owner and user. I had wanted to take all his belongings home with me, but common sense prevailed and I selected some items and placed them in a box. I picked out the clothes that he had worn in his final days; they still bore the scent of his favourite soap. I took some photographs of Dad in his younger days and a couple of books. I also took Dad's clock and his watch; somehow, these time-pieces were important-my time with him ended the moment he went over that ledge.

As I was leaving, I caught myself glancing back, hoping to see Dad at the door, sending me off, a routine that he had maintained for many years. No matter how tired or weak he was, he would insist on seeing me off even if he had to use his walking frame. I glanced back one last time but he was not there to wave goodbye, a painful reality check. I left the apartment with his life in a box and a heavy sorrow in my heart.

The drive home was filled with thoughts of Dad, his death by suicide, and how much I missed the exemplary father who had brought me up. Had he not been such a good father, I might not be missing him so much. I might have been spared such a deep and raw pain. The drive home also triggered painful memories of the times when he was in the passenger seat next to me. As I drove on, it dawned on me that I would never have him in my car again. I did not realise that his mere presence in my car had been such a source of contentment and security for me. I cried bitterly at the thought that I would never be able to enjoy his company again.

upon reaching home, I placed my box of Dad's belongings in the study. Each time I went into the study, I felt an immediate connection with Dad simply because his things were there. I needed to hold on to that bit of connection. But it was also a very powerful trigger of raw emotion. Eventually, I decided to put the box away in a less conspicuous place, a place I could go to each time I wanted to revisit the memories of him; a place I could avoid if I felt emotionally fragile.

Flashbacks and intrusive thoughts

Every day, every hour, every moment when I was not thinking of something else, the events of that fateful day kept replaying in my mind. I cried for Dad and for myself. Whenever I had some time to myself, my thoughts would drift towards Dad and his suicide. I recalled the drive to Dad's place that morning and our last conversation. Repeatedly, even when I did not want to remember, I could almost hear myself say goodbye to him that day, and his wistful last word to me, "OK. " I wondered why I did not detect the difference in his response. Dad would normally say more than just "OK" whenever I said goodbye to him. He would always tell me to drive carefully and remind me not to speed; and he would always nag me to have my meals regularly knowing that I suffered from gastric pain. Why did I not notice this short, sad reply?

I found myself counting the days and feeling that they were slipping by too quickly. I wanted time to stand still and, if possible, take me back to the day when Dad was still alive so that I could do something to prevent him from taking his own life. I wanted to be transported back to the days when I was able to hold him up from his sleeping position so that he could be fed, so that I could talk with him, to show that I cared and to assure him he was not alone even though he was experiencing great pain.

My thoughts about Dad were especially vivid when I was alone. I was constantly plagued by unrelenting questions that yielded no answers. Why did Dad take his own life? What was going through his mind before he jumped? What were his last thoughts? That phone call from my brother about Dad's suicide kept coming back to me, followed by the shock and guilt I had felt. I kept berating myself for not being more alert, for not picking up the signs of distress, for not doing more. Why didn't I stay longer that day? There was nothing that I had to do that afternoon that was more important than keeping him alive. Why didn't I chat with him a bit longer? Why didn't I realise the significance when the maid reported that the day before his suicide, Dad, despite his weakness and frailty, had insisted on walking to all the windows in the apartment? On hindsight, it became clear to me that he was choosing his spot.

Guilt and remorse

I was racked with guilt whenever I thought of how I had failed Dad. I failed to take good care of him, protect him, and to ensure that he lived happily in his old age so that he could return home to God peacefully. There were endless ruminations of "should have", "could have" and "if only". It was sheer torture brooding over the various alternative endings. But I could not help myself. The "if only" scenarios buzzed in my mind whenever I failed to keep myself preoccupied with other matters.

If only I had stayed with him that afternoon, he would have been alive. My presence would have prevented the tragedy. If only I had detected the depth of the hopelessness in his voice. On the many occasions that we talked, he had mentioned his desire for God to take him home. He did not want to be a burden to anyone. If only I had told him how important he was in my life and how much I needed him to be around as long as possible. I had erroneously believed that the constant care and love of his family would see him through these despondent moments in his life. When he spoke of returning home, I knew that he was serious, but I had not realised how desperate he was to end his life on earth. I did not realise that he was contemplating suicide. He had always been a positive person and in spite of his depression I clung stubbornly to the hope and the belief that he would somehow survive the low period in his life, since he had always been resilient. If only I had invited him to come live with me so that I could spend more time with him. Maybe that could have assuaged his feelings of hopelessness and he might have felt less neglected. If only I had cut down on my other commitments, I could have freed up more time to spend with him. Perhaps that would have lifted his spirit and he might not have chosen suicide. I was so busy helping other people; perhaps I had neglected Dad.

If only he had been able to get adequate rest he might have been less depressed. I should have taken his complaints of insomnia more seriously and be more willing to administer stronger sedatives. I was reluctant to give him heavier doses of sedatives lest he overdose. And if I had not been so focused on pre-empting an overdose, perhaps he might still be alive.

To deal with the guilt, I visited Dad's niche every week. I would stop by the florist, choose Dad's favourite flowers and proceed to where his ashes were kept. I would clear out the previous posy of withered flowers and place the fresh ones in the vase. Whilst doing this I had little conversations with Dad in my mind. I would tell him how things were with the family and particularly how the children were faring in school. Dad was proud of his grandchildren's academic achievements. Whenever my children did well in major exams, Dad would encourage them further by giving each child an ang pow.

The trip to the niche was inevitably wrought with memories of Dad and how he died. For many months I visited Dad's niche every week. It was my way of dealing with the burden of guilt that I was carrying. It was also my way of maintaining some form of connection with Dad. I remember missing him to the point where my heart ached.

As Mum's niche was next to Dad's, the reality that both my parents were dead and gone forever could not have been more stark. I would usually leave the place in tears and with a heavy heart. If only I could be given a second chance, I would definitely do things differently. Sadly, there was no room for bargaining; there could never be a second chance; death was final and nothing could be done to reverse that.

I went through periods of analysing or trying to analyse what went wrong. "Why did it happen?" "How did things go so wrong?" "What could have been done to prevent the suicide?" I was fully conversant with all the 'if only' scenarios, and yet, they did not lead to any satisfactory answers. In my desperate need to have some sort of answer that made sense, some sort of certainty, I took to blaming others for Dad's suicide.

Triggers

Dad's death coloured the ordinary things and everyday tasks that I had taken for granted. Numerous sights and sounds took on a new meaning and triggered a fresh wave of grief. Whenever the telephone rang, my heart jumped; I recalled the times when Dad called just to chat with me. Everywhere I went in my own house, there were memories of his visits. It also became difficult to drive past places I had taken him to. Since it was impossible to avoid them, I frequently found myself peering at the road through a continuous stream of tears. Driving became synonymous with crying and I became adept at doing both simultaneously.

There were some triggers that I could anticipate and avoid. In those early days I took pains to avoid walking past the barbershop that I used to take Dad to for his haircut. I had to put away the DVDs that Dad had enjoyed watching at my home. There were also songs (his favourites) I could not bear to listen to. And whenever I saw an elderly man that vaguely resembled Dad in his later years, there would be a lump in my throat. These I had anticipated.

But some triggers took me completely by surprise and I didn't know I would be affected until I found myself crying. On one such occasion, I was in the wet market buying fresh fish when the fishmonger asked me why I was buying so little that day. It was an innocuous, factual question because my weekly order usually included Dad's portion. I choked up with tears, mumbled an apology, and hurried off.

Family and friends

The first few months following Dad's funeral were tough. It was also very trying for my husband and children. I did not want to talk about Dad and his death because I could not come to terms with the fact that he had taken his life. I tried to suppress most of my negative thoughts and feelings; I told myself that I was doing this to protect my family members from having to deal with the pain and grief that I would not be able to control if I brought them out in the open.

It would have been easier to recall past memories with fondness if Dad had died of old age or sickness. However death by suicide was different. How does one anticipate and prepare for a suicide in the family? I was not prepared when it happened; and after it happened I was not prepared to talk about it. In many ways it was almost unspeakable because there were no words to fully describe the horror of the event, the magnitude of the loss, and the depth of the grief.

What I could do was cry; and I cried and cried everyday. There was no telling when the tears would flow. My husband, a sensitive man, was often at a loss for words when I cried. He wasn't sure how to comfort me. Fortunately for me, he did not press me to talk; instead he would simply hold me tightly.

Sometimes, instead of tears I became uncharacteristically impatient and snappy. My husband bore the brunt of my outbursts.

The children were not spared. They were quiet and seemed to be walking on eggshells in my presence. There were times when they tried to cheer me up, but they were largely unsuccessful. I knew that they were struggling with their own grief and sadness just as I was with mine. But I was not ready to broach the subject with them. I was fearful of questions that they might ask; questions that I could not answer. I was especially apprehensive of the 'why' and 'how' questions. How do I even begin to talk about their grandfather's suicide? How do I explain why he took his own life? I lacked the courage and emotional energy to face these questions and to provide comfort to others in the family. So I busied myself with busyness and buried my grief in silence, convinced that this was not a good time to talk about his death, that I should not trigger intense sadness for the family by talking about it. And the family took their cue from me.

We talked about everything except Dad's suicide. The family became adept at skirting round the topic. It became the elephant in the room that everyone saw but pretended was not there.

Anger and blame

I battled with anger almost daily; and each day I lost the fight to control the intense negative emotions raging in me. This was the toughest struggle in my journey towards healing. In my head I knew that it was no one's fault that Dad chose suicide as a way out of a painful existence, but rational thinking took a back seat as I pinned the blame on my siblings, the maid, the doctor, and finally, even God.

As much as I was angry with myself, I was also angry with my siblings for what I perceived to be their neglect and failure to care properly for Dad when he was ill. I felt that they too did not treasure Dad enough to give him the care he deserved. He had given so much of himself to us, his children, and yet we did not do enough when he needed us most; when he was at his weakest. Our collective efforts fell short of what was needed to keep him alive. But I did not want to create a scene; Dad would not have wanted that. So I had to suppress my anger and maintain some semblance of family unity however superficial. As far as possible I avoided seeing or meeting up with my siblings for fear that my body language might betray my anger towards them. When such family meetings were unavoidable, I had to work hard to contain my true feelings. I was restrained in my conversations with my siblings as I carefully steered away from any possible talk about Dad or his suicide. I was not confident of managing my emotions and was very fearful that any conversations about Dad's suicide might arouse the anger within me and I might explode with hurtful and unfair accusations that would tear the family irreparably apart.

I was extremely angry with the maid. Of all people, she was in the best position to avert the tragedy that day because she was present and it was her job to check on him. Instead she was taking a nap when Dad jumped. That nap cost Dad his life, cost me my father and my family. Dad died on her watch. If she had not been asleep, Dad would still be alive. I could not bring myself to talk to her in the days following Dad's suicide because I knew there was no way I would be able to hold back my angry words.

I was angry with Dad's geriatrician for not doing more to help him. Since he could not speak Dad's dialect, he spoke to us instead.

If Dad had been able to get direct assurances from the doctor, perhaps that might have been enough to give him hope and to tip the balance in favour of living.

Sometimes, my anger was non-specific. It was directed at the healthcare institutions in general. I blamed the system forthelong wait to see a doctor whose consultation would last mere minutes. Advice and prescriptions were dished out without any consideration as to the difficulties the family might have in keeping the patient safe. Where was the empathy that should underpin every healthcare service? Why didn't the doctor or nurses try to find out what was really troubling the patient and what might provide some relief? Was that too much to ask? I was also angry with society at large, for everybody's careless attitude towards the infirmed elderly.

I was so angry, so irrationally riled, that even God was not spared. Dad had been a church-going, God-loving Christian all his life; he kept the faith despite the hardships in his life. God could have prevented this tragedy from happening. Why didn't He intervene? What had Dad done to deserve this? Or was God trying to punish me? If so, what wrong had I done?

Was I angry with Dad for the decision he made? But how could I be angry with him when I had witnessed his suffering? In many ways, I could empathise with him. It was obvious that he lived until it became too painful to live any more. In a way, I could fully understand his desire to end the pain which could not be diminished by medicine or prayer. In all honesty, I was not angry with Dad as such. But there were times when I felt upset with him for leaving me with the pain of losing him in such an unbearable way, for making me a survivor of his suicide. Dad had been a survivor of suicide himself; he had had a first-hand experience of the heart wrenching agony a survivor had to go through. So a part of me could not understand why he resorted to suicide too. Didn't he realise that I would be left to struggle with this incomprehensible and unmitigated sense of loss?

It was my nature to respond phlegmatically to difficult situations. So it was excruciatingly uncomfortable for me to contain such strong negative and disturbing emotions. I also did not know what else to do to cope with the turmoil that seethed within. I felt off-balanced and did not know how to restore the equilibrium that I was accustomed to; I did not know what I could do to bring relief. Since I could not express the anger, it morphed into a dark sadness that sat in my heart. Life felt meaningless.

I found solace in solitude. The beaches at Changi and East Coast were my refuge. The angry waves crashing onto the sand and retreating from the shore reflected the turmoil in me. It soothed my grief without taking it away.

Double tragedy

My grief journey was complicated by something that happened many years ago. Dad's suicide excavated the thoughts and feelings which I could not or did not know how to express when my mother died. You see, Mum also died from suicide. I was still in primary school when it happened, and I don't remember feeling much at that time. But now, 40 years later, the pain of that first loss returned and weaved itself into the grief over the loss of my Dad.

On the surface, my family seemed quite normal, with a father, a mother, two brothers and me. But life was anything but normal when Mum was alive. My strongest memory of her was of a tired woman who was physically present but emotionally absent. She retired to her room for long stretches of time to sleep or just to stare out of the window. She was apparently on medication which made her sleep excessively. When she was awake, she seemed detached, oblivious and passive. It seemed to me that my Mum did not bother to interact with me or to get to know me; she was lost in her own world and I felt neglected. I did not know then that she was suffering from depression.

I wanted a different mother, like my neighbour's mother, someone who cooked and cleaned and took good care of the family. In my family it was Dad who shouldered these responsibilities. However busy he was, I sensed that he was always there for his sons and especially for me. He took care of our needs and attended to our growing pangs and emotional problems that Mum should have catered to but did not.

In addition, he also had to take care of Mum who was repeatedly admitted to hospital for attempting to take her own life. On those occasions, he would explain that Mum had to go to hospital because he could not wake her up. Each time it happened, I would be left on my own because he had to be at the hospital with her. I resented that. I could not comprehend my Mum's multiple suicide attempts. But I remember feeling fearful, bewildered and abandoned byher, and worried formy dad who had to dash between hospital and home.

Mum tried to die so many times that it was only a matter of time before she finally succeeded—through an overdose. She went to bed and slept through the afternoon. Dad could not wake her up. I heard him calling her name again and again, but she did not stir. I saw her lying on her side facing the wall. Dad must have called the ambulance. I don't remember what happened after that. But this time she did not come home from hospital. Dad explained that she died because she had taken too much medicine.

I don't remember feeling especially sad about losing her because I was more absorbed with my Dad's well-being. Her death by suicide brought great sadness and pain to him. I saw him cry and it frightened me. Nobody had explained the grief process to me, so in my childish mind I concluded that tears were a sign of weakness and an inability to cope. At the funeral, I made sure that I was constantly at his side to remind him to stop crying. I had lost my mother and I did not want to risk losing my father too. I needed him to be strong. And if tears were a sign of weakness then my task was to make him happy. I remember the many 'what if' and 'if only' questions that he used to ask me in the weeks after Mum's suicide. I listened although I did not understand what he was going through. All I knew was that I needed to be vigilant so that the sadness did not get to him, so that the sadness would not take him away from me. I monitored his moods, I kept him company when he looked lonely, and I did what household chores my childish hands could manage in the hope of providing him some relief. My brothers kept themselves busy with their own activities outside the home.

Dad's continued presence provided all the security I needed as a child, and since I did not enjoy a close relationship with my mother, I did not really miss her during the couple of years after she died. It was only when I was into my teens that I began to feel the loss. I did not miss her per se, but I sorely missed the presence of a mother. However hard he tried, Dad could not be a mother to me. For example, I became conscious of the changes in my body but there was no one I could turn to for advice or comfort since I was the only female in the household. I was completely unprepared for my first menstruation and Dad had to ask the lady next door to teach me what to do. My friends and classmates seemed happy and carefree and well adjusted; and I attributed their well-being to the fact that they all had two living parents to guide them. I felt inferior to them. I was envious of my friends and angry with my Mum for her absence, for my emotional deprivation and low self-esteem. But I felt bad about feeling angry with her; after all she was sick.

Somehow I stumbled through my teenage years. But the loss resurfaced when I became a mother myself. Once again I found myself having to cope without the benefit of an experienced presence to guide me on the finer points of motherhood. I envied my friends who had mothers who stayed with them during their confinement period. Their mothers cooked special confinement food, and helped mind the baby so that they could rest. I felt sorry for myself because I had to manage on my own; a motherless mother.

It was only much later, in my 30s, that I really began to miss Mum, the person who died in my childhood and not just the idea of a mother. By then I had read some books on depression, and even had friends who were depressed, so I began to understand some of the challenges she must have faced. I still felt sorry for myself, but I also started to feel sorry for her. The parallels in our situations also helped me to empathise. My Mum was a stay-home mother; she had three children and had to manage without any help from a maid. I had also become a stay-home mother with three children; but even with the help of a maid there were times when I felt overwhelmed, exhausted and lonely.

Looking back, I wished that I had known her better. I longed to hear her talk about herself. I wanted to know what she thought, how she felt and what she endured. I wanted us to have a mother-daughter connection that I could cherish. I did not dwell much on the fact that she had taken her own life because it seemed so long ago, not relevant any more ⋯ until Dad, too, decided to commit suicide.

As I grieved for my dad, I became increasingly aware of my Mum's suicide and it compounded my sense of abandonment. Why did God allow both my parents to die this way? Why my family? Why me? Why?

Stigma and shame

If Dad had died of illness or old age, I would have had no hesitation in disclosing that information to relatives, friends and well-wishers. But in this society, death by suicide carried a stigma which was difficult to ignore. And I found that I was not impervious to what others thought. Like other survivors, I needed to save 'face'.

Before Dad's death, I had an extremely shallow understanding of suicide. I could not fathom why anyone would resort to taking his or her life. Yes, living could be tough, but whose life wasn't? I felt then that people who chose to die through suicide had opted for an easy way out; they were cop-outs, selfish and self-centred people who had no regard for the pain that they would inflict on their loved ones. I was certain that others held such views as well which influenced me to keep Dad's suicide a secret. I did not want people to think less of him because of it.

I also felt ashamed that Dad's death was through suicide, and not ill health, old age, or even accident. The relative at the wake who accused me of being uncaring, convinced me that I would be judged by others, either to my face or behind my back, that relatives and friends would conclude that Dad had been neglected and felt unloved, which drove him to suicide. My own reputation was at stake. And I did not want people to think less of me.

The stigma and shame associated with suicide made it difficult for me to reach out and get support for myself. I belonged to a church community that provided support to its congregation but I could not bring myself to discuss Dad's suicide with my pastor and church members. Instead, I withdrew from them to safeguard my shameful secret. I was fearful that disclosure would only bring scorn, avoidance, morbid curiosity, and other negative responses. At best, some might have been sympathetic and reach out to me out of Christian duty. But I did not want to be an object of pity and duty.

In much the same way, I kept away from many of my friends to avoid being disappointed by their responses too. Whenever I considered confiding in them, I would be filled with questions I imagined they would ask, and I would change my mind. How should I explain that my love and care were not enough to make my dad want to continue living in spite of his pain? How could they understand that I had done my best but it was not enough to make Dad choose life? I could not make sense of Dad's demise through suicide, much less explain it convincingly to others.

Given Dad's advanced age, friends simply assumed that he had died through natural causes. I did not deliberately set out to lie but I did not do anything to correct their assumption. Even then, people's lack of sensitivity amazed me. Some were quick to try to provide comfort by reminding me that Dad had lived to a ripe old age so there was really nothing to be sad about! Others spouted meaningless platitudes and condolences. I became adept at pretending that I was coping well; I smiled and accepted their condolences graciously. But behind the mask of calmness and control, I felt like a fraud.

Because of my secret, the support I had was limited to a few friends who were privy to the truth. But even with the best of intentions they sometimes inadvertently made unhelpful comments. I was mortified when one of them tried to comfort me by comparing my grief with those who had lost their spouses or children to suicide. My loss of an aged ailing father to suicide was apparently deemed less horrendous than the suicide of a spouse in the prime of his life or the suicide of children who represented our future. And therefore my grief was expected to be shorter and less painful. This line of reasoning totally disregarded my close bond with Dad.

Helplessness and hopelessness

Each morning, I would wake up wondering what I should do to keep the sadness at bay. When Dad was alive, his needs would take up a lot of my time and energy. Taking him to the doctors and doing his marketing were my routine chores. All of a sudden, Dad was gone and with his death, I was left not only with time, but time to dwell on Dad and how he died. A heavy sense of dread engulfed me as I wondered how to go on living when there was such a deep cavity in my life that others around me just could not fill.

How did life become so fragile and transient? He was alive in the morning and in the blink of an eye he was gone in the afternoon. Just like that, life was snuffed out. During those initial months my life was practically devoid of meaning. I felt that his death had robbed me of the joy of living, and without joy there was a sense of hopelessness, and without hope, life felt meaningless. It seemed that there was nothing for me to look forward to every day. I felt hopeless and helpless, both for myself and the impossible situation I was in. If life was full of nothing but intense sorrow and mental anguish, what was the point of living? Yet life had to go on. But it was difficult to wake up in the morning knowing that I would feel low and lousy.

Some nights I dreamed of my dad as he was when he was alive. I have since forgotten most of the dreams; perhaps I did not want to remember because remembering brought fresh grief. But one particularly poignant dream has etched itself permanently in my memory. In this dream, Dad telephoned me to ask why I had not spoken to him for such a long time. The dream was so real, it made waking up so unbearably painful that I cried.

In the initial three months of mourning, I felt overwhelmed. On many occasions, I found myself bursting into tears whenever I thought of or talked about Dad. I found myself swinging from an eerily quiet sadness to sudden outbursts of anger, and there were times when I was especially unreasonable

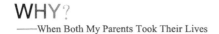
towards those who were close to me. Perhaps their love for me made me feel safe enough for me to vent my frustration and misery on them. But it did not ease the horrible ache in my heart. My family still needed me to see to their daily needs, but who was going to see to mine?

Chapter 3

Who Helped Me

I expected life to gradually return to normal, except without Dad. But three months after his suicide, I found that I was not feeling any better. Physically, I could manage the housekeeping and parenting chores, even the social engagements that came with being a wife and a member of an active church community. I could also continue my volunteer work at a hospice. But I felt exhausted and I could no longer manage my grief which manifested itself in uncontrollable crying spells. I cried in the car, I cried at home, I cried on the streets, I cried at restaurants with Tina, I cried in church. Everywhere I went I was reminded of Dad; the places I had taken him to, the meals we had together, the way he had looked and the things he had said to me. And every time my memories were triggered, tears flowed. Crying provided some relief, but it did not last and soon I would be overwhelmed with tears again. I was feeling stuck, worn out and discouraged. And most of all I felt all alone and empty. Talking about my feelings with Tina made me realise that I had to do something. I could not carry on like this.

Tina must have reached the same conclusion because she gently coaxed meinto seeing acounsellor at the Samaritans of Singapore (SOS). She heard that in addition to working with people who were contemplating suicide, SOS was also working with the loved ones who were left behind.

Getting help

I resisted her suggestion because of my pre-conceived notions of counselling. I thought that counselling was for people who were needy and psychologically weak. I saw them as wimpy or whiny types who could not cope and needed someone to tell them how to live their lives. I could not imagine why anyone would want to talk to a stranger who was after all just another human being with his or her own struggles and problems. What could this stranger do that family and friends could not? I thought of myself as a balanced person and that there was no problem too difficult for me to manage especially since I had a healthy network of friends and family. Horrible though it might sound, the thought of seeing a counsellor made me cringe. So the whole idea of me needing counselling help was absolutely preposterous.

My impression of people who called the SOS hotline was similarly skewed. On the one hand, they had my sympathy because they were in distress and must have been in great need since they did not mind talking about their problems to strangers on the telephone; I thought of these callers as lonely and friendless people who did not have family and friends they could turn to. On the other hand, there was a part of me that wondered why they did not try harder to develop and maintain family relationships and friendships. Had they done so, they would have had little need to call the SOS hotline and depend on the support of strangers.

Yet I did not know what to do with these tangled feelings. My husband and children were supportive in their quiet ways; they were always available when I needed company and gave me space when I needed to be by myself. But I could not talk to them about my deeper feelings because I did not want to alarm them with my dark thoughts. I did not want to cause them more anxiety. Tina had been a wonderful friend; she texted and called me daily, and once a week we lunched from noon until sometimes as late as 5: 00 pm. I could speak more freely with her but I feared that the constant focus on my issues and my needs would wear her down. She graciously assured me time and again that she was not tired of hearing me talk about my grief, but I was getting tired of hearing myself talk repeatedly about my situation. Moreover, as my best friend and someone who was acquainted with my family, it was difficult for her to be impartial. She had her own opinions and there were times when I would have welcomed an objective perspective. So when she suggested seeing acounsellor, I seriously began to consider it. We talked about it over several lunches.

I agreed that it might be helpful to talk to someone else who could remain objective and help me to sort out my thoughts and feelings about Dad's suicide. I told myself that in some sense, it might be easier and safer for me to express my feelings to someone who was a stranger to me. I convinced myself that I should be able to share honestly and openly since counsellors are supposed to keep things confidential. Tina assured me that whatever I said would stay within the four walls of the counselling room. I also thought that it might be helpful to see someone who had been working with suicide survivors and was familiar with their struggles. And as Tina put it, I had nothing to lose because I could stop going if it did not work out.

Arriving at the decision to contact SOS was not easy, but implementing that decision seemed like an even bigger step. I sat at my desk at home. It was a weekday and no one was around. I had the telephone in my hand and was hesitating to punch the SOS numbers. I had always been the volunteer helping those less fortunate, but there I was on the verge of becoming a person in need. I felt very sorry for myself. After a long hesitation, I dialled the SOS number, punching the digits one at a time slowly, and even then, I was in two minds about whether I was doing the right thing. A couple of times I stopped dialing halfway and thought long and hard about what to say to the person on the phone. And then I started again. Twice I managed to dial straight through but I remained silent when the phone was picked up and I hung up because I was not ready to speak to the person. On the fifth attempt, I finally found my voice and made an enquiry about their support group for survivors — the Healing Bridge. I was asked to wait while she got the person in charge to speak to me.

I was instantly struck by the lady whom I spoke with: her voice exuded warmth and kindness. I felt at ease almost immediately. She answered my queries patiently and spoke unhurriedly. She asked when I had become a survivor and whom I had lost. Because she sounded very kind, assuring and understanding, I broke down in tears. Even then, the silence was not awkward as she waited for me to regain my composure. I readily accepted her invitation to come to SOS to meet her. She seemed to understand the turmoil in me. At the end of the conversation, I felt relieved. And yes, I was also grateful for her invitation to meet her. That conversation gave me hope. I had found a professional who had worked with survivors. I had found a counsellor I could connect with. The person whom I spoke with was the late Mary Mathew, then Executive Director of the SOS.

One journey, two counsellors

When the date of my appointment with Mary drew near, I started to have cold feet. I had no clue as to what would transpire during a counselling session and what was expected of me. I wondered what Mary was like in person. Would the person match the voice I spoke to or would she be different in person? If Tina had not offered to accompany me to my first counselling session, I might not have turned up at all.

We rang the doorbell outside the black wrought-iron gate at the entrance of SOS. I felt self-conscious to be in a place that provided help to the desperate and suicidal. What if I bumped into someone I knew? What if people thought that I was suicidal too? At the very least I would be perceived as being needy. By coming to SOS, I was acknowledging that I was in need of help. The helper had become the "helpee". It was a humbling experience and the first of many which helped me to be less proud of my own ability to cope and to be more understanding of those who ask for help.

I was ushered into a room, a square-ish space just large enough to hold three armchairs and a side table which held two boxes of tissue paper and some pamphlets. There were no windows so no one could peer in. I gratefully accepted an offer of a cup of tea. Even today, whenever I think of that first session with Mary, I would remember how the cup of tea helped put me at ease.

Mary was tall, slim, and exceedingly gentle. She listened attentively as I spoke about Dad's suicide. I surprised myself at the ease with which I opened up to her. It was easy confiding in her even though the recounting was painful and made me cry. Her presence was a comfort and for the first time in many months, I felt that I was no longer alone because here was someone who understood and asked questions that helped me tell my story. My initial hesitation and anxieties about seeing a stranger was no longer a big issue. I agreed to return for follow-up sessions.

At our second meeting, I was extremely touched when Mary herself shed tears as I spoke about the pain of losing my dad. Her tears communicated empathy and her willingness to journey with me. She took me through the events on the day of the suicide to help me heal. Mary used her questions skillfully and sensitively, like a surgeon slicing open the purulent wound to drain the pus. The pain was excruciating. But she did not send me home with an open wound. She dressed the wound with kindness, warmth, concern, empathy and even tears. These gestures were like balm to an infected wound and a wounded soul.

I cried so much during these sessions that I usually went home with a headache. I remember needing to sleep off the exhaustion as soon as I arrived home. We met fortnightly, but some days I was reluctant to see Mary because of the pain of remembering and talking. It was easier just to keep busy and suppress the pain. There were friends who wanted to catch up with me over lunch, errands to run, the house to be put in order, and my children and husband needed attention. It was tempting to make the excuse that I could not spare an hour every two weeks for counselling. Ironically, now that I had found someone I could talk to, I found myself thinking of ways to avoid talking because this kind of talk was more painful than talking to Tina. But a part of me knew that the healing would take longer if I postponed the counselling. Though the sessions left me emotionally and physically drained, I had a gut feeling that healing was somehow taking place because I no longer felt as hopeless as before. I was hopeful that with Mary's professional help, I was going to feel better in time to come. My sessions with Mary were a concrete step in that direction.

As it turned out, I had only four sessions with Mary. During our third session, she was visibly in pain whenever she had to sit down or get up from the chair. Her back was hurting but she managed to remain focussed and attentive. I remember telling her to take care of her back and to take her time in sitting and getting up. After our fourth session, Mary went on long medical leave. Somebody from the office called me to cancel my next appointment with Mary. I did not know that she was not coming back. Perhaps she did not know either. She died of cancer ten months later, about a month after Dad's first death anniversary. I learnt of her demise from an article in The Straits Times that featured her work in SOS.

I attended Mary's funeral with an extremely heavy heart. I saw many people at the funeral and wondered whether like me, some were her clients who had also been touched by her words of kindness. The hymns sung at the funeral and even the eulogy triggered memories of the funeral for my Dad a year earlier. Her death was another blow to me. I came to her mourning the loss of my Dad and Mum, and ended up mourning for her, too. I could not understand why God had allowed her to suffer an illness that would end her life prematurely and deny people the help that she could give. I did not have the courage to attend the cremation service because I could not cope with the memories it would stir up in me. My brief encounter with Mary left an indelible impression on me. She was The Good Samaritan who gave me the courage to enter the pain of my loss and to begin my journey as a survivor. She had touched me at a point in my life when I was in greatest need. It was a tremendous blessing to have met Mary.

When Mary had been on medical leave, I was told that someone else would take over as my next counsellor. I was extremely reluctant to take up the offer. I felt that no one could take Mary's place and I did not want to repeat my story to anyone else; it would be too tedious, onerous and painful. I was unsure whether my next counsellor would be a good fit for me and I had many doubts.

Would she be as warm and kind as Mary? Would she also be as gentle? Would she be a good listener? Would she be able to help me to express my thoughts and feelings? I thought that perhaps it would be the perfect time to bid SOS goodbye. I told myself that the four sessions with Mary had sufficiently healed me and I should now be able to get on with life. Opening myself to Mary and losing her so suddenly and prematurely had left me feeling vulnerable. I did not want to go through that again. Worse, I did not have the chance to repay Mary for her kindness. It was a debt I could not repay.

I told myself that I should be able to manage now, to get over the pain, to somehow skip over it, just keep busy with all my commitments and I would be fine. Busyness would be the panacea. I began to keep myself fully occupied with no time to feel sorry for myself. I made sure that my diary was filled with social and other engagements so that I would not have a moment to myself. My role as chauffeur to my three girls kept me on the road several times a day and, in between, I met friends for breakfast, lunch or tea, and took on more volunteer work at the church and the hospice. I moved from one activity to the next, making sure I had no free time because any free moment would inevitably lead me to think of Dad and his suicide. I suppressed my feelings to keep myself from falling apart. It did not work. I became physically unwell and I experienced anxiety attacks. For no apparent reason, my heart would beat faster and I became very fearful for nothing. I was getting worse, not better. It became clear again that I needed professional help. So reluctantly, I called SOS and asked to see the counsellor who was supposed to take over from Mary.

Ophelia was totally different from Mary. That made it difficult for me to warm up to her initially. Mary had a disposition that was similar to mine; she was quiet and subdued. Mary used to sit back and sip her coffee. I had my cup of tea and we sat like two friends except that we were in SOS. Ophelia was more animated. She leaned forward when I was talking and she used her hands for emphasis when she asked questions. I could tell that she was trying hard to engage me. But she had a more difficult task of eliciting responses from me because I was still missing Mary and I was reluctant to be drawn in. I was also reluctant to repeat my story as a survivor because it meant revisiting the pain of my loss. But Ophelia persevered and so did I. As it turned out, I went back to see her for another 30 sessions over one-and-a-half years.

Mary and Ophelia were also different in their counselling styles. Mary was more micro whereas Ophelia was more macro in her counselling approach. Mary would pick up details as I shared and would then focus on these details. At times, the whole session or most of the session would be spent on one particular aspect of my story. She would listen intently like a friend as I talked. Ophelia was more active. She attended to the challenging issues that I raised and would ask questions that would invariably lead me to my own answers. Sometimes it seemed that she intentionally asked questions that had no answers, but these questions made me think and raised my awareness of my thoughts and feelings as a survivor. I could tell when a question was coming because her brow would furrow up as she thought about her questions. After several sessions, I began to warm to her and my trust in my new counsellor gradually grew. I even looked forward to my sessions with her. I found that we spoke a common language using analogies and metaphors. Sometimes she also picked up pen and paper and drew what we had been talking about. Those images and analogies helped me to understand my experience of suicide grief. Eventually, I was able to confide in her quite openly and with a candidness that surprised even myself.

I am describing the differences between my two counsellors not for the purposes of deciding who was the better counsellor, but to highlight the need for both counsellors and the counselled to persevere despite differences in personality and approaches. Both Mary and Ophelia were exceptional counsellors and I had the fortune, or misfortune, of being counselled by them. Had I the choice, I would have preferred not to have needed their help and service. But I also know I was lucky to have them counsel me. My time with these two empathetic, conscientious, and caring counsellors helped me immeasurably in coping with Dad's suicide. Coming to SOS was one of the wisest decisions I made in my journey of grief.

One of the things that I have learnt during my sessions in SOS is that each survivor is unique. We have our own way of grieving, there is no right or wrong way of going about it. And we have our own way of recovering and readapting to life. What worked for me might not necessarily be helpful for the next survivor. But here are some of the things that I was able to take away from my counselling sessions at SOS.

Metaphors for healing

In one session, I talked about my anger, guilt, frustration, sadness and bewilderment. I felt that these and other feelings were all tangled up inside me like a ball of wool. I felt helpless because there were just too many feelings inside of me; I could not even name some of the feelings I had, and I did not know what to do withthose I could identify. I am the sort of person who is particular about things being in their proper places. I like things to be organised, including my thoughts and feelings. At home, I am always straightening things and putting things back in their designated places. And here

I was walking around with what felt like a total mess inside. Picking up on my analogy, Ophelia suggested pulling out the threads one by one and dealing with the tangled mess one thread at a time. It was such a simple idea and yet it gave me a sense of control over the mess. The message I received from this analogy was that my feelings, however painful, could be dealt with one at a time, with some help.

And then she surprised me by asking me what I would do with the threads after I had untangled them; did I see myself knitting the wool into something which I might store away but bring out occasionally to remind me of Dad? This metaphor started me thinking that perhaps I could make something good out of the bad thing that had happened to me. It jolted me out of my helplessness, and made me realise that although I had no control over what had happened to me, I did have some say over what to do with my experience of the tragedy. It was also a good reminder to be patient with myself because knitting (and healing) takes time.

One constant metaphor we used was that of a survivor being thrust into taking an enforced journey into unknown terrain. How could I not feel daunted by the prospect of having to be on a journey alone especially when the destination was unknown? It was normal to be dealing with a lot of uncertainties because of the special nature of the journey. I was not sure how long my journey of grief would last and whether I could survive the rough terrain. But at least I had some idea that this would be an extraordinary journey and it was normal to feel anxious about it. It put things in perspective for me. No wonder I was feeling overwhelmed and helpless. I was also able to use this metaphor when I wanted to reflect on my experience as a survivor. The initial part of the journey had been the most challenging and frightening; I did not know where I was and I could not see what was ahead of me. It was very hard for me to imagine I could even begin to feel better. But after I started getting help from SOS the journey became less arduous. For the first time since Dad's suicide, my heart felt lighter and I could discern some hope on the horizon.

Subsequently, when I joined the support group for survivors, I was comforted to know that I had fellow sojourners with me-some ahead, some behind and others walking alongside me on this journey of grief.

The metaphor I liked best came up when I lamented that Dad's life did not end well. He had been a good father to me; why did he spoil his life with such a tragic ending? Ophelia asked me to think of what it would be like if Dad's life story was described in a book. How many chapters would there be? What would be in these chapters? I envisaged 10 chapters of wonderful reading, an engaging and inspirational account of a devoted father, but chapter 11 ended the book with a tragedy. I liked the metaphor because it suddenly dawned on me that there were 10 good chapters. I could choose which part of the book I wanted to read and re-read. I had good memories of my Dad. I did not have to dwell on chapter 11 all the time.

I remembered these metaphors in particular because these were the ones that sustained me in between sessions and whenever I was feeling down.

It's OK to cry

Going for counselling meant talking about the pain of losing Dad which usually ended up with me in tears. Tears are therapeutic. They are necessary for healing. But the connection between tears and healing is not obvious when you're the one sobbing and wailing. My knowledge that crying is therapeutic did not fit with my initial experience of it. In some ways, crying provided relief because it let out the pent-up pain. But it did not feel like I was healing. Instead I felt exhausted, broken and fearful that I might not be able to pull myself together again. It was also embarrassing to be reduced to that level of helplessness—weeping in front of a stranger. It shattered my self-image as a prim and proper woman with a reputation for providing comfort to others.

The crying made me dehydrated and gave me a headache and I had to sleep it off after each difficult session. And there were times when I wanted to give up counselling altogether because, contrary to my expectations, counselling was actually making me feel worse. What kept me coming back was my confidence in my counsellor and her repeated reminders that it would get much worse before it got better. She would end the session by telling me "You're going to feel worse after seeing me. " She was right. So I learnt to adjust my expectations. But it gradually got better. The tears gradually washed away the rawness of my grief. I also found that I was less prone to crying fits outside the counselling room, having cried buckets during counselling.

At home, I would cry only when it would not attract too much attention, and as far as possible, not in front of the children. I also tried to control my tears when I was out with well-meaning friends, though without much success. But at SOS, I had a safe place to cry and I could cry as much as I wanted to. Crying in the presence of a counsellor also meant that I could get support and comfort without taxing my loved ones. Over time, crying became therapeutic; my sobbing became less intense and I began to feel lighter.

It's OK to laugh

Laughter, too, was therapeutic. It might seem strange to associate laughter with suicide grief counselling, but there is a role for the appropriate use of humour. Laughter produces endorphines, a neurotransmitter produced by the body, and used internally as a painkiller. It also gives us a natural high without the use of artificial substances like drugs, alcohol and food, among others. My counsellor had a great sense of humour and she used it with respect and sensitivity.

I have always enjoyed a good laugh. You would not suspect it looking at my petite frame, but I have a bellyaching kind of laughter. However, after Dad's suicide, I could not get myself to laugh again. I even felt that it was not right for me to laugh again; that to laugh or be happy again would be an indication that I did not love my Dad enough. I felt that I should be in a state of perpetual mourning instead as proof that my love was not shallow or transient. But Ophelia would sometimes say something that made me laugh. It surprised me that instead of feeling guilty, I felt good. One of our private jokes centred on my persistent request for a progress report on my recovery as a survivor. My counsellor jokingly threatened to bring in a chart at our next session so that we could track my weekly progress; I laughed when I realised how ridiculous that sounded. I was trying to track my recovery as if it were a stock market phenomenon.

Sometimes it was not her intention to make me laugh but laughter came anyway. One such occasion was when I moaned that I felt Dad's absence most on Saturdays because that was usually when I would spend a lot of time with him. Ophelia observed that I still had 7 days in my week but they were now Monday, Tuesday, Wednesday, Thursday, Friday, Sadday and Sunday. The simple act of re-naming my Saturdays as Saddays made me laugh. I think the laughter came from my relief in discovering that my suicide grief had made me different and yet in some ways still the same as other people. In accepting the renaming I was giving myself permission to feel sad on Saturdays, and I had no expectations that others would understand because this was my version of a Saturday, not theirs.

When I could laugh again, it also became easier to forgive myself. Ophelia would gently tease me about my need to control everything. It somehow helped put things in perspective for me. Certainly I could have done better in caring for Dad. But life this side of heaven could never be perfect no matter how hard I tried to control the outcome of situations. Moreover Dad would not have wanted me to shut all laughter out of my life because of what he did. So I learnt not to kick myself all the time. Sometimes it was enough just to laugh off small mistakes.

It's OK to get angry

The anger that I had suppressed in early months now made its presence known in ways I had not anticipated. I thought l was managing to direct my anger at the weeds in my garden. My idea of gardening had always been to enjoy the sights and scents without lifting a finger. But after Dad's suicide, I would attack the weeds to vent my anger which had no other outlet. Apparently, that was not enough; it needed other targets. One unfortunate bank official became a convenient target when my anger spilt over. I scolded and shouted at him in the course of discussing a financial product. Everyone at the bank turned to look at me. That behaviour was so out of character for me and especially over a small issue. It was the first time in my life that I had raised my voice that way.

I also felt angry during the counselling sessions. For a while, I wondered what this anger was about, until I realised that I was angry with myself for needing to depend on a counsellor to help me cope with my loss. This did not sit well with me, especially since I felt that she was helping me because it was her job and not because she wanted to. My access to her was constrained by appointments. I wanted very much to be able to just pick up the phone and talk to her whenever I needed to, but that was not possible because as long as she was counselling me, she was not allowed to be a friend whom I could contact as and when I needed to. Mum's and Dad's suicide had magnified my sensitivity to being abandoned, and I felt angry with my counsellor for not being available outside of her working hours.

I was also angry with Ophelia for her seemingly detached demeanor. She seemed unaffected while I felt extremely broken and shattered. There were times when I would be sobbing intensely, tears streaming down my face while she looked calm and unfazed. She empathised with me, but in that room I was the only one hurting and that made me mad.

We talked about the anger I felt towards my siblings and repeatedly, I asked what I could do to end that struggle. Finally, she asked, "What would it be like for you if you did not get a chance to forgive your siblings?"

I was taken aback, and became very upset with her for suggesting a solution I did not ask for and I left the session perturbed and frustrated. The next day I called and told her about my anger towards her. She listened and acknowledged it and even apologised for not hearing my needs accurately. My anger dissipated.

In the course of volunteering at the hospice, I had read some books on grief and I knew that anger was one of the five stages of grief according to Elizabeth Kubler ross in her book *On Death and Dying*. But I did not expect anger to be so uncomfortable and unreasonable. And yet, to heal, I had to allow myself to understand and express that anger.

It's OK to talk about the same thing again and again

I had a great need to talk about Dad and I repeated my story over and over to Ophelia. Tina also received a good measure of my repetitive lamentation and reminiscing. But I did not talk much to my husband or children because it was my way of protecting them. They tried hard to cheer me up and I did not want to disappoint them by presenting them with evidence of my ruminations.

It was easier to reminisce with Tina because she had met Dad and my family. But there was a limit as to how much I could impose on a friend, albeit a close one. I was more willing to share with my counsellor because she was a professional listener and there was less danger of my burdening her. Most of my one-sided conversations centred on memories of Dad, the time we spent together, and his many good attributes. I also talked a lot about missing him and my feelings of remorse and anger. But I imposed limits on myself because I did not want to bore her or be long-winded. So I reached a stage where I would not mention the same things unless she asked. Thankfully she asked about the same issues at our sessions and I was able to talk about missing Dad again and again.

I would have liked to be less repetitive, but I felt compelled to tell my story over and over. repeating my story felt good because it purged it from my system and allowed me to put it out there where it could not hurt me so much. It also reassured me that it was not my fault. Slowly, the ache weighed less heavily and constantly on my heart and mind. Sharing my story with a counsellor who had worked with other survivors was clearly an advantage. Ophelia regularly assured me that retelling my story was an important and necessary part of healing. So I talked and talked until I no longer felt the need to talk about it at length or in such intensity and frequency.

It's not linear and it's not the speed that counts

When my counselling began, I thought that if I attended my sessions faithfully, I would be rewarded with progress. I had expected the grieving process to be a straight line starting with the trauma and ending with the healing. I expected to feel less sad after each session, and after a couple of sessions I ought to be able to manage on my own again. Speed was of essence because I wanted to wrap up the grief work quickly, get rid of the counselling crutch, and get on with my life. I was even preparing to migrate so that I could start life anew for myself and my family. Perhaps in a new environment there would be fewer triggers and fewer sad memories to haunt me.

But I was the only one with the timeline. Ophelia told me that I would be feeling worse, not better, after seeing her. It was true. I felt a lot worse before I began to feel a little better. But I did not give up on my timeline for recovery. After a year of counselling, I felt ready to say goodbye to her. So at our next session, I shook Ophelia's hand and thanked her. Then I made an unsolicited donation to SOS to make sure I did not leave behind any debts of gratitude. Now I was ready to migrate. Or so I thought.

Barely two weeks later, I found myself calling SOS to make another appointment. I was feeling depressed and needed to talk some more. returning to SOS was a setback to me and I was sick with disappointment. Ophelia reminded me of the close bond I had with my Dad. Since he was such an important person in my life, would it really be possible to get over this loss so quickly? How long had I known him? All 47 years of my life. How long did I give myself to "get over it"? I had thought that one year was a long time for recovery but against a lifetime of knowing him I realised that I might never get over it. If I migrated I would leave the physical triggers behind—the sights that usually evoked sad memories of him. But what would I do with the memories that I carried in my heart and mind? Would I be able to leave them in Singapore too? I knew then that I could not rush through the grief process. My pain is a testimony of my love and it would not do justice to his memory if I tried to distance myself from that pain as quickly as possible.

That was when I realised my life would never be the same again. It would never be normal again in the way that it had been in the past and that I would have to adjust to a different life. It was not just a different life without Dad—I had been made different by my experience of losing Dad through suicide.

My grief process was like a never-ending spiral that touched the same issues, feelings, thoughts, memories again and again. Sometimes the intensity of feelings decreased and then it came back with a vengeance. I have come to expect this "return" particularly on festive occasions. The first Christmas without Dad was especially difficult. I felt his absence keenly and was hardly in the mood to celebrate. Traditionally, Christmas had always been celebrated in my home and I had always looked forward to hosting the occasion. I felt that I could not cope with celebrating Christmas since it would only remind me that Dad was gone forever. But I remembered that Dad had wanted all his children to be together as a family. So with a heavy heart, I went ahead with the celebration, all the while feeling empty and sad. The Christmas lights and carols everywhere seemed so incongruent with the loss and darkness I felt within me. After Christmas, there was Chinese New Year to get through. By the time Christmas came around again, I noticed that I was still missing Dad and the longing and emptiness were still there, but they were no longer as excruciating as I expected. There were also times when I thought I was done with anger and it resurfaced though less overwhelming and debilitating than in the early days. The pain was never again as extreme as it had felt in the beginning.

When I stopped trying to get over the grief I could accept and embrace the reality of my loss better. The grief did not take up so much space in my heart when I gave up the struggle to kick it out. There was room for other memories to return. The loss of Dad through suicide is a part of me now; I carry it with me wherever I go and whatever I am doing. But I am also carrying treasured memories of a gentle man and a loving father.

Chapter 4

What Survivors Do

It took me more than a year, after Dad's suicide, to experience the benefit of mutual support through the Healing Bridge, a group started by the SOS for survivors of suicide. Although I had enquired about the Healing Bridge in my first call to SOS, it was just my way of starting the conversation. I was not really seeking to be part of a support group for various reasons, some of which only became clearer to me as I started writing this chapter. Perhaps other survivors can also identify with the reasons behind my initial reluctance.

Crossing the bridge

Even though Mary had told me that the Healing Bridge would be the place to go to talk about my struggles and receive support from other survivors, I was dead set against it. I valued my privacy more. Only a few close friends knew about Mum's and Dad's suicide then. Even my pastor and my church community were not privy to this information. So I could not picture myself sharing my private thoughts with a group of strangers. It was hard enough sharing with one stranger—the SOS counsellor. It was unthinkable making myself vulnerable to so many.

Before Dad's suicide, I knew nothing about support groups. From books and TV shows, I thought they were groups of people sitting in a circle and talking at the same time, dominated by those with the loudest voices. They seemed extremely needy and met week after week with no fixed aim except to share their dramatic stories. I wanted no part of it.

I was also fearful of meeting someone I knew at the Healing Bridge. Word might then get out that Dad had committed suicide and I might have a lot of explaining to do-that it was not due to my neglect, which would seem defensive on my part.

I felt no reason to join a support group because, apart from Tina, I was already getting good support from my sessions with Mary, and subsequently Ophelia, who were generous in making time whenever I asked to see them. Neither pressured me to join the group.

Only as I was writing this did I realise, to my dismay, that another major reason for my reluctance to join the Healing Bridge was my pride. Perhaps, I was reminded of my childhood years of having to depend on the charity of others when Dad's small business failed. The family had to move to more affordable lodgings and that was when Mum's depression seemed to have started. Those early days of hardship created a phobia of having to depend on others. Even the thought of seeking help from a professional counsellor was abhorrent.

On reflection, I must have also feared the inevitable emotional pain of sharing my experience. Or worse, my own pain would be amplified by the stories of other survivors. Their suicide stories would bring on more sadness and sorrow than I could manage. It did not make sense to be constantly reminded of Dad's suicide when what I wanted was to leave it behind.

So how did I end up in the Healing Bridge? The turning point came a couple of months after Dad's first death anniversary. After abortive attempts to terminate the counselling sessions and migrate, I was still seeing my counsellor. I became increasingly curious about how other survivors coped. Did they have the same struggles with guilt and anger? Did their pain and longing linger on too? I did not wish to be the only one still whining one year after the suicide. How did they manage special occasions when families gathered for anniversaries, birthdays, Christmases, Chinese New Years? I wanted to know whether they were also fearful of such occasions. My feelings were not as raw as they were a year ago and I felt more ready now to meet other survivors and listen to their experiences.

My counsellor told me that there was someone in the group who had also lost a parent to suicide. I thought that this person would understand what I was going through. Who else would understand what it was like to lose both parents to suicide? Non-survivors may not appreciate fully the struggles of coming to terms with the suicide of a loved one and the pain that lingers long after. Ophelia was able to help me understand some of my experiences and feelings but she was not a survivor herself; no matter how much she empathised, she could not possibly fathom my pain.

I also had this nagging thought that by now I would surely have outstayed my welcome with close friends who had been listening to me talking about the same thing again and again without much apparent improvement. A support group could offer fresh support since my grief was taking a long time to wear off.

The passage of time had also lessened my fear of bumping into friends or acquaintances in the Healing Bridge meetings. Or perhaps I was better able to think more clearly. Since the Healing Bridge was only for survivors, perhaps they, too, had the same reservations. Moreover, I felt emotionally stronger and to some extent, ready to disregard the opinions of those who did not understand. Or at least I felt that I had enough courage to try.

I also joined the Healing Bridge with something of a Messiah Complex; I felt a strong desire to be there to help fellow survivors. Perhaps it was my way of trying to make sense of my parents' suicides. I felt that I was coping better and I wanted to help newer survivors, to be of some use to them, so that I would not be just receiving help all the time. So when Ophelia mentioned the support group to me again, I said yes.

The first meeting

As I drove to my first Healing Bridge meeting, I was apprehensive. I wondered what kind of stories I would hear and what effect these stories would have on me. I was afraid that all the intense, negative feelings I had in the initial period after Dad's suicide would resurface and I might be overwhelmed by grief. I felt alone and regretted not having Tina with me. Although I had, by now, made my own way to SOS on numerous occasions for my counselling sessions, I felt like I was going for the first time all over again. Every u-turn sign on the road was a temptation to drive off in the opposite direction. It was raining heavily and traffic was bumper to bumper—a perfect excuse for me to call the SOS office to tell them that I could not come. I clung tightly to the steering wheel to make sure that I did not back down. When I arrived at the SOS premises, I took my time parking the car before gathering enough courage to approach the main entrance. Even then, I lingered outside for a while, before finally pressing the doorbell. One of the staff opened the door and then I was in. There was no turning back.

I heard the laughter of my fellow survivors first, before I met them face to face. I had come in feeling apprehensive and expecting a serious and even depressive atmosphere; their laughter seemed out of place. I couldn't see myself laughing on such a serious occasion.

I was ushered into the SOS training wing which also served as the Healing Bridge meeting room. Ophelia was there with two survivors, who came forward and shook my hand when she introduced me to them. Lian and Joanne had both lost their husbands to suicide and had been survivors for about two years. I was impressed that they had not just survived, but done well in their recovery. Healing had taken place to the extent that they were able to co-facilitate the Healing Bridge sessions with the SOS staff.

We had tea and refreshments and made small talk as we waited for the others to arrive. Among them were those who had lost spouses, siblings, parents and children. When the session started, Ophelia reminded us of the need to maintain confidentiality so that everyone could share freely without any fear that their stories might become public. As each survivor shared his or her story, tears flowed freely as some of us cried for ourselves and for each other. We were grappling with our pain as individuals and as a group of people who understood what it was like to lose a loved one to suicide.

When it was my turn to speak, I felt a lot of sadness again but there was also a sense of relief. There was no false hope that the pain of my loss would go away through talking. I knew it would stay with me for the rest of my life, and would at times be more acute. My experience was similar to that of the other survivors. I felt safe there, sharing the pain of my loss. No one judged or condemned me because we were all survivors. I could not share freely with my family members as I had wanted to protect them from my pain and to spare them from worrying about me. But I could talk freely as part of this group who understood and empathised with my grief, and that gave me a sense of belonging. To my surprise, members gelled quite quickly from the first meeting. The camaraderie was palpable despite our different faiths and backgrounds. I had expected that the commonality that existed among us would cause us all to bond at the same level and with equal intensity and closeness. However, it was not the case, as every individual was different and there were those who were more drawn to some than to others. I needed to temper my expectations. I went away from the first session feeling emotionally raw but relieved that I finally got to meet other survivors. The six sessions came to an end just when I felt that the bonding among members was getting stronger. Members exchanged phone numbers so that they could contact each other when they needed to talk about their grief. I was grateful when my new friends from the group sent me messages of support and told me to telephone them if I needed to talk.

Since then, I have attended four rounds of Healing Bridge over two years.

And each time there were new survivors joining the group, each with a personal story of loss and suffering. The survivors who have been in the journey longer usually led the way with their sharing. Their presence was a source of comfort and strength to the newly bereaved, and a clear indication that it was possible to survive the tragedy of suicide.

The survivors

Talking about my pain and loss and listening to stories of fellow survivors made my journey of grief more bearable and a lot less lonely. Although my sessions with Ophelia were crucial for my healing, she would eventually move on to coach someone else as I moved ahead in my journey. My relationship with survivors was different. We shared a commonality that made us fellow sojourners. With them, I could take my relationship to a deeper level. I could also call on fellow survivors whenever I needed someone to talk to. Any illusions I might have had about being alone in my pain was dispelled by the stories I heard. Here are some of the survivors' stories that made a deep impression on me (To protect their privacy, I have changed their names and personal details.)

Sheila

Sheila's mother had suffered from depression for many years before jumping to her death from the common corridor outside their flat. I felt a special affinity with Sheila because of the similarities in our situations. Her aged mother ended her life in the same year and month and in the same way as my aged Dad. Sheila was also the only girl in a family of boys, and she had a special bond with her mother just as I had with my Dad. Her mother's struggle with depression reminded me of my Mum's illness. As Sheila described her mother's lethargy and loss of interest in all activities, I began to understand better what my own mother must have gone through. With Sheila, I mourned the loss of a special bond with a parent, and through Sheila's story of her mother's depression, I began to understand my Mum's behaviour in a way that made more sense than just reading about depression in books.

Sheila shared her story with much sadness and tears. She sounded extremely tired. Like me, she was having a hard time attending to her own needs as well as those of her family. At home her children did not want to see her crying as it made them feel insecure. Whenever she cried, her four young children would try to stop her by comforting her and insisting that she played with them. I understood her children's behaviour because when my Mum committed suicide, I did not allow Dad to cry. I was worried that Dad might be overwhelmed by grief and would also resort to suicide. I was constantly by his side, ever ready to comfort or distract him whenever he was feeling sad. As I shared this part of my story with the group, I began to realise I had had to grow up before my time. It was a heavy burden for a child to be responsible for her parent's safety. Perhaps that would account for my somber demeanour as a child. Opening up and sharing about that episode in my life brought a lot of pain and I remembered leaving the room in tears, being emotionally overwhelmed. The painful memories of myself as a little girl were too much for me to bear. I was petrified of going into pieces in front of the other survivors. Ophelia followed me out of the room to ensure that I was not alone. That gesture meant a lot to me as it reinforced what I knew all along: though the journey would be excruciating, I was not alone. Looking back now, I realise that there was no need for me to leave the room. It was OK to cry with my fellow survivors.

Sheila also spoke of conflicts among her siblings after her mother's suicide. The pain of her mother's suicide was compounded by the loss of good family relationships. The same thing happened in my family. Although there were no open conflicts in the aftermath of Dad's suicide, I felt, somehow, that relationships with my siblings were strained, and that things were not the same and would never be the same again for my family.

I was inspired and encouraged by Sheila as I observed her journey. She had attended one round of Healing Bridge the previous year. So this was the second round for her. Though the pain of her loss was apparent, she was willing to talk openly about her on-going struggles. Though she was grieving, she reached out and comforted the other survivors seated near her. When I saw her again at her third round, I heard her describe her coming to SOS for the Healing Bridge as "coming home". It was here that she could share freely with us about her mother. She said that we were like family to her. At one of these sessions, she came wearing some gold bracelets that had belonged to her mother. What had previously been difficult for her to even look at was now a way of maintaining some connection with her mother.

I felt so encouraged by her that it motivated me to visit my brother's apartment where Dad had spent his last years. Hitherto, I was very afraid of seeing the place again and revisiting the painful memories of Dad's last day. I had not been back since the day I left with a box of Dad's belongings. Going back was a personal milestone for me. I went straight to Dad's room. His bed was bare, his cupboard empty. I cried as I recalled his presence in that room. Then I went into the dining room. His favourite chair was still there. I had sat beside him many times at this table as he had his meals. And finally I looked at the window he had jumped from. I wept. I looked back one last time and finally shut the door to the apartment and felt a sense of closure. I had overcome my fear of being there.

Joanne

Joanne struggled to put her life together again after she lost her husband to suicide. He had been suffering from depression for several months. He was getting psychiatric treatment but he did not feel any better. On their wedding anniversary, she rushed home after a frantic call from her maid and was told that he had jumped from the bedroom window.

By the time I met her at the Healing Bridge, she had been a survivor for two years. It was her laughter I heard when I came for my first Healing Bridge session. I did not know then that behind the laughter was an ongoing struggle to hang on to life, for the sake of her two girls. Each time she shared her story, I could sense how isolated and lonely she felt. She had become a widow and a single parent overnight, on top of having to handle the financial and practical matters that her husband used to take care of. unfortunately for her, her parents were not as supportive as she had expected them to be, and her in-laws blamed her for not taking better care of her husband. She felt very betrayed and abandoned by him. She had done everything she could to reassure him and provide him with emotional support. She could not understand why he gave up when he had said he would not. She could not understand why he left her when he had said that he loved her.

Joanne felt the loss of her spouse most keenly whenever she took the children out and they saw intact families walking or eating together. At such times her younger daughter, who was home when her father jumped, would poignantly ask,

"How come I have no Daddy?"

Her questions became more persistent when she started primary school and the class talked about families.

I admired Joanne especially for her courage in sharing her experience openly with the group. She spoke her mind, and her feelings showed in her choice of words and her tone of voice. Her presence was particularly helpful to new survivors because she helped us feel comfortable in the group by sharing her own thoughts and feelings, however negative or painful. She made it possible for us to talk about our negative emotions too. She also talked about struggling with her own suicidal thoughts. There were times when she wanted to give up and would have jumped-if not for the support of Mary, her SOS counsellor and subsequently the Healing Bridge members who kept in touch with her and reminded her to stay alive for her children.

Joanne's story helped me to understand how devastating it was to lose a spouse to suicide. The loneliness and abandonment she spoke of was echoed by other survivors who had also lost their spouses. Still, she was willing to talk about it. When I first heard her story, I was struck by her honesty. The anger she felt towards her husband for leaving her to take care of their two girls was very raw. But these days, it surfaces only when she has difficulties coping with additional stress from work. He was the one who had attended to her and calmed her whenever she had a bad day at the office. After his suicide, he was the one she vented on.

"When I'm OK, he can rest in peace," she would say, "Otherwise, I will scold and curse him. "

Joanne said that she would never be happy again. But she tries to make her children happy by taking them out even after a tiring week at work, and making time for holidays with them. Every now and then, her eyes would sparkle as she joked mischievously with the other survivors. Joanne is a firm believer in the support that members of the Healing Bridge can provide because of their shared experiences. She believes that healing can take place in a group setting.

Jascintha

Jascintha lost her only son to suicide. Her story made me think that surely nothing could be as painful as the suicide of one's child. Her teenager had been receiving treatment for depression when he decided to jump from a block of flats. She had cooked his favourite food and was waiting for him to come home that day. He never did.

She joined the Healing Bridge about four months after her loss, so her emotions were still very intense. She burst into tears when it was her turn to share her story. At home, she was unable to talk about her son because her husband and two adult daughters did not want to talk about their loss with her.

They knew that she was in deep grief and did not want to add to her pain. And she, too, suppressed her crying to protect her daughters.

Jascintha blamed herself for her son's suicide. She felt that, had she been a better mother, he might still be alive. Many things in their home reminded her of her son. The sight of his slippers made her wonder whether he was still around. For a fleeting moment she allowed herself to believe that maybe he had not died after all. She had left his room untouched and would often go into his room to lie on his bed. I cried with her as she described how she tried to capture his presence and his scent by hugging his pillow and smelling his tee shirts. She talked about his cheekiness: the way he used to tease her, the way he played with his pet cat and other triggers which brought back painful memories. Her son's cat was both a comfort and a painful reminder of its master. She could function at work, but whenever she came home, she had no energy to cook or do the housework. Yet before the suicide, she would wake up early every morning to do housework and prepare meals before she left for work. Now she felt very tired all the time because she had not been able to sleep well after her son's suicide.

After my first run, the group dispersed and I did not see Jascintha when I returned for the next run of the Healing Bridge four months later. Two of her relatives had since passed away and the family was once again in mourning. But I will always remember the chicken stew she cooked and brought to the group in the final session, and the way she beamed when we complimented her cooking.

Gan

Gan's younger brother had some problems at work. He became depressed before finally ending his life by jumping from a block of flats. Gan felt angry at his brother for not thinking of the effect his suicide would have on the family.

"Even if he has no feelings for me, a brother, how can he do this to his mother and father?" he would lament.

Gan came to the Healing Bridge to find out more about depression. He wanted to understand the cause of his brother's suicide. Most of all, he wanted to learn ways of preventing other suicides in his family. He regretted that he did not have a chance to get to know his brother better. His brother had kept to himself and did not confide in any member of the family. Gan had tried to assure him of his support whatever the problem, but his brother did not respond. He wanted to make sure that henceforth, everybody in the family would communicate better. Apparently, communication in the family had become worse after the suicide. In his enthusiasm to learn more, he was prepared to do some reading until he realised that all the books in the Healing Bridge library had been written by foreigners. No local survivor had written about their experiences. Part of the reason I decided to write this book was to address this need.

And yes, men do cry. I was touched by Gan's openness in sharing his helplessness. Gan cried as he talked about his failure to save his brother and his desire to prevent another tragedy in his family. He was determined to make things better for his family but, as a survivor who had been in the journey longer, I wondered whether he wasmovingtoo fast. Ifeltthat heshouldgive himself more time to grieve the loss of his brother, before focussing on solutions.

Mr. & Mrs. Wong

Mr. and Mrs. Wong had no idea that their young adult son had been troubled, so it came as a complete shock when he killed himself. Of their four children, he was the one they had been least worried about, since he had always been independent and capable of looking after himself. When I met them in the Healing Bridge, they had been struggling for three years. It was still unbearable for them to think of packing away the belongings of their deceased son. They shared how well-meaning friends and relatives had been urging them, "It's been so long, why don't you move on?" was one typical refrain. But it was hard for them to move on because whenever they met their nephews, their colleagues' children, and other young people, they were always reminded of what it might have been like if their son were still alive.

They were struggling very hard to come to terms with the fact that they had lost him and their future with him. They coped by supporting each other, through psychiatric consultation and lately, through SOS counselling. They also attended the Healing Bridge. Like other survivors who come in with another family member, they were placed in separate groups to give each of them the space to talk about their grief—without constraints and without having to worry about the effects of their sharing on the other family member. This was one place they could express their grief without being told to move on.

Nothing can ever prepare us for the loss of a loved one through suicide, but when it happens, it helps to know what to expect. The return of good memories comes later but in the meantime, we have to get through the fatigue, the fears and the facades.

Fatigue—the importance of self-care

During the Healing Bridge sessions, I noticed that the new survivors always looked more tired and drained than those of us who had been there longer. They looked like they had not slept well; their eyes were lifeless and heavy and ringed by dark circles. Their whole body sagged under the burden of their grief. Several talked about being unable to sleep, others felt aches and pains in various parts of their body, and they fell sick easily. Yet they continued to work themselves hard and kept extremely busy to ward off the grief.

The same thing had happened to me earlier. Every part of me was under tremendous stress. My chest had a dull ache. The first couple of nights, my mind was in overdrive thinking about the suicide, so I could not sleep. Physically I was bone tired, but I could not rest as there were many matters to settle which seemed more important than resting. I even purposely kept myself busy with activities to cope with the grief, which added to my fatigue. I was trapped in this vicious circle, unaware that it was wrecking me physically and emotionally.

I also did not eat much because I never felt hungry. One day, a friend commented on how gaunt I looked. My bathroom scales showed that I had lost three kilograms over a couple of months. I ignored these warning signs of exhaustion because I thought I was all right.

During one of my sessions with Ophelia, she remarked on the amount of time and energy I was devoting to volunteer activities in the hospice and in the church community. She advised me to slow down and not spread myself too thinly. She often said I should take better care of myself before caring for others. I would listen politely to what she had to say, but I never took her advice seriously. I would even roll my eyes (only in my mind of course) as I despised the thought of self-care. To me the needs of people around me were tremendous, and there was so much that I could do to help alleviate their pain and suffering. Self-care reeked of selfishness and self-centredness. I certainly didn't need it, I thought, especially when I felt that I was managing my time and commitments well. Whatever Ophelia said about self-care went out of my head the moment I stepped out of the counselling room.

The concept of self-care was alien to me because I grew up taking care of others. It had been that way since Mum's suicide made me the only girl in a household of three men. From the age of seven, I had helped Dad with household chores and I became his caregiver because there was no one else as relatives avoided our family after the suicide. So Dad looked after us and I looked after Dad. Years later, when I was studying overseas, I was constantly looking out for fellow students from different parts of the world. I helped them settle down by providing emotional and practical support. The pattern continued when I returned to Singapore. It was natural taking care of others even when I was busy, first with work then with being a wife and mother.

I did not take care of myself until a major anxiety attack about seven months into counselling. That really frightened me. I did not want to resort to medication to help me manage further attacks, so I finally heeded Ophelia's advice and slowed down. I took a break from volunteer work at the hospice, and I reduced the time I spent giving emotional support to friends and church contacts. Drawing boundaries around myself gave me some time for myself. But that meant I had periods of "unbusyness" when I feared that my depressing thoughts would recur. To cope, I started taking regular walks, sometimes with friends and sometimes by myself. My appetite picked up and I was able to eat and taste food better. I started reading for leisure-books and magazines that I did not have time to read before. Not just books on death and suicide but also novels and inspirational works. Ophelia taught me some deep breathing exercises which were helpful whenever I felt anxious. Stopping whatever I was doing and just focussing on my breathing had a calming effect. I also started a journal so that I had someone to talk to very frankly in between counselling sessions.

Grieving is hard work, and it took me a long time to recognise this. using busyness as a form of self-care to cope with my grief was effective only for a short time. While it helped initially to keep me occupied and distracted from thinking about Dad, it could and should not be used as a long-term coping tool.

Fears are normal

I did not mention this to friends, but after Dad's funeral, and when life became routine again, there were moments when I felt alone and fearful. I kept thinking about Dad's suicide. I could not control those recurring thoughts and I feared that I was going bonkers.

I was relieved to hear that the other survivors in Healing Bridge had their share of fears too. In fact we all had very specific fears. Joseph related his fear of heights. His mother had jumped down from his apartment andbecauseof this, hewouldbe seized by fear and his knees would go weak whenever he looked out of his apartment window. He would have to hold on to something to steady himself. This fear of heights as an adult was totally unexpected. Gan's constant fear was that he might lose other family members to suicide. So he regularly lectured them to communicate if they had problems. Nick said that he was fearful of medication. Following his father's suicide, he had seen a doctor to help him manage his grief. Medicine was prescribed, and though they were helpful, he was afraid of them because his father had been treated for depression in the same way before his suicide.

So there we were, adults admitting that we had all these irrational fears. As I listened to them, I realised that I was normal. It was clear that none of us were crazy. Having thoughts of going crazy was normal for a survivor.

Secrecy and privacy

One of the first things we learn to do as survivors is to "wear a mask", as one Healing Bridge member puts it. Choo said that he had to pretend that he was coping well because of his unpleasant experience with friends who avoided him. They did not want to hear about his wife's suicide again and again. They were supportive when the suicide occurred and during the wake and funeral. But they wanted him to move on after that. As a result, whenever he went out with them, he had to pretend that he had moved on. Likewise for Joseph whenever he was with his colleagues. They would talk about everything except his mother's suicide. And he followed their example. The Wongs who lost their son to suicide had to pretend to be fine at home so as not to upset their other children and their elderly grandfather. Whenever the Wongs felt their grief rising to the surface and threatening to overwhelm them, they would step outside to cry.

Aside from sparing our friends and family our pain, we also wear masks to protect ourselves from the scrutiny and judgment of others. I guess, in the context of Asian society, "face" is very important. Although I would like to think of myself as more enlightened, the shame of having a suicide in my family made me keep it a secret from many people. I had to remind myself constantly that Dad's suicide was not because of me. I had done my best to care for him though I was not always patient and understanding. Gradually, over the past two years, I found the courage to tell a few more friends the truth about Dad's death. Sometimes, I still said that he died of old age. Having to lie did not sit well with me and I would feel guilty. But I think I will continue to lie to most people because they do not need to know. Not because I am still ashamed and need to keep it a secret, but because Dad's suicide is a private family matter. For this reason too, I decided to use a pseudonym for this book, to respect my family's right to privacy and to spare them unwanted attention. But I use my own name when I am with survivors or talking to survivors. I do not know whether my brothers had talked about Dad's suicide with their friends; somehow I doubt it. So the last thing they need is media publicity.

It makes me angry whenever I see a suicide story sensationalised by the media. I was lucky to be spared media coverage but Joseph was less lucky. The press hounded him for weeks until he had to disable his door bell and stay away from home for long periods.

Hurtful comments

Sometimes, perhaps unwittingly, people can be cruel or insensitive when they talk to survivors. Some remarks by relatives, friends and acquaintances are not only unhelpful, but damaging as well. This issue surfaced repeatedly during the Healing Bridge sessions. And it affected both new and veteran survivors.

I remember that at Dad's wake, one day after his suicide, a relative concluded that Dad had taken his own life because I did not offer to take him into my home. I felt extremely hurt because her remarks suggested that I was responsible for Dad's action. Her remarks seemed to validate my own struggles with self-blame and my feelings of guilt and remorse. I rushed to the toilet and cried.

Other survivors suffered equally from thoughtless comments.

One survivor who had lost a son was told,

"At least your case is better than those whose children are missing."

Joanne's friend said to her,

"It's been several years already; why don't you find yourself another man?"

After six months of watching Mr. Wong grieve for his son, his boss instructed him,

"I want you to stop grieving and get on with life".

At first I thought that it was just outsiders who did not understand because they were not in our shoes. But even survivors could make such remarks. Sheila's sibling could not bear to see her crying so he told her,

"Die already, cry for what?"

An acquaintance of mine, who had lost her husband to suicide, told me that losing her husband was "more painful than you losing a father". She was not a Healing Bridge member, and thankfully, none of my group members had ever uttered such unkind words.

Sometimes, the remarks are not intended to hurt and are simply common greetings on festive occasions. But it can be painful for a survivor to respond to "Merry Christmas", "Happy New Year" and "Happy Birthday". As Joanne put it,

"What is there to be happy about? I will never be happy again."

Hardly surprising, some survivors like Lian choose to be out of the country during festive occasions to avoid these happy greetings and the family gatherings, when relatives with their complete families would make her feel the absence of her husband most keenly.

Perhaps people are sometimes at a loss as to what to say and in trying to fill the silence in the conversation, they talk without thinking. Or perhaps they are just clumsy in conveying what they mean. It is also possible that they are exasperated with the survivor's repetitive reminiscing and whining. There will always be people who will make such remarks for whatever reason and motive. These remarks deepen the pain of the survivor. Some survivors choose to avoid insensitive people or ignore the remarks of those who do not understand the feelings of a suicide survivor. I have found it helpful to talk about these hurtful remarks with a friend.

On my journey with other survivors, what struck a chord in me was their willingness to share their stories, honestly and openly, to heal themselves and help others come to terms with their loss. Yes, coming to the Healing Bridge has exposed me to tragic stories, but it has also opened my eyes to the resilience of the human spirit. This I have learnt: It is possible to overcome tragedy and rise above suffering.

Chapter 5

Where Is God?

I could not pray.

I did not choose this journey;

It chose me, I had no say.

Oh God, why did you Let him die that way?

I could not pray.

The shock, the truth,

The shocking truth of what was said.

Oh God, where were you When my father died that day?

How could I pray?

No comfort left for me.

First you let suicide take my mother;

Oh God, was my lesson better learnt

When it also took my father?

How could I pray?

Left standing here in naked sorrow

Bereft of hope and branded;

Oh God, did you see me,

And did you feel me bleed?

Oh Lord,

I am so weary,

I walk alone, I am in need.

My words are full of anger

But my soul is full of grief.

Oh Lord,

Somehow you heard me,

Or was it me who did not see

For when I looked again

With your grace I saw relief.

With outstretched arms

They held me

And journeyed with my fears

And hand in hand we're walking

Though our path is marked with tears.

I do not know, I'll never know

Why this painful journey chose me.

But I thank you God

For those you sent To walk this journey with me.

Throughout this ordeal, one question plagued me: Where was God in this tragedy? A year-and-a-half later, I was still struggling and would continue to struggle with it. Writing about it had been equally difficult, especially concerning my anger with God and His response. Or the lack of it.

Although I was never a fervent Christian, confronting God became part of the journey of grief. Writing about God now is also my way of thanking God for holding on to me when I felt utterly helpless and hopeless.

My parents were Christians and I was brought up with Christian values. These values were caught rather than taught. Dad did not talk about Christian love or his relationship with God, but somehow, he demonstrated this love for God. He was a helpful man and a good neighbour. There were times when he willingly minded the neighbour's children when they needed a babysitter. On numerous occasions, Dad offered to pick up groceries for our neighbours. And when they were sick, he helped out any way he could. What made an impression on me was that he extended help not only to people with in the church community, but also to those who were not of the same faith as he. He was a patient man, gentle and kind, and rarely lost his temper. I would come home from school with bad report cards that had many negative comments from the form teacher and grades written in red, indicative of poor results. Dad would sit down, look at the report card and grades, sign his name and tell me to try harder next time.

Although Dad practised Christian love, strangely, God was not real to me. Dad might have had a relationship with God that motivated him to demonstrate Christian love, but it was not the case for me. I was trying to find the reality of God in my own life. Dad did not or was not able to articulate God and His teachings in a way that I could understand intellectually. Looking back, I needed to know more about this God that I was supposedly worshipping, and why He deserved my worship and adoration. The Bible taught that Adam and Eve sinned and, therefore, I needed God's forgiveness, but I wondered what their sin had to do with me. I had no idea what the gospel meant. Therefore, going to church on Sundays became a weekly routine that held no spiritual significance for me. At times it was fun, other times boring, and most of the time meaningless. Good Fridays and Easter Sundays were reduced to bunnies and eggs. Christmas was little more than an occasion for food and fun. Looking back, I realised that the adults in that church, including my Sunday school teachers, did not talk about God in a way that was meaningful to me. They did not explain to me the inherent sinfulness of Man and the reason Christ had to die on the cross. Perhaps they, too, had difficulty articulating their faith and belief in God. But I continued to attend church out of obedience to my Dad.

In my teens, I continued to question God and religion. An idealistic, angst-ridden teenager, I decided that no one was going to force me to go to church. Not even Dad. My Mum's suicide when I was a child had caused me to feel different from my friends. Her suicide, though not as devastating as Dad's, nonetheless had made me envious of families that were intact. I also felt inferior because of my family's dire financial situation. People from Dad's church would come by with petty cash. Instead of giving the money to Dad in private, some of them would make a show of their generosity without any thought to his feelings. I detested that. Dad was in no position to reject their charity. He would look miserable and visibly upset, especially when the money was given to him for all and sundry to see. To me, these Christians were not walking their talk; the help they extended was borne out of a sense of duty and not love, and perhaps even motivated by a need to show how generous they were. If love was the hallmark of Christianity, I certainly did not see or experience it. I did not want to identify myself as a Christian or be part of the church. To my Dad's dismay, I decided I did not want to go to church just because I had to; it should be because I wanted to, and I did not want to anymore.

I stopped attending church in my late teens. Looking back, it was necessary for me to have those "desert wandering" years. Away from the formal teachings and setting of the church, I started to think about God, and what it meant to have God in my life. There was an emptiness within me which I could not understand. I felt that there should be more to life than going through the daily grind of study, sleep, eat and play; of being born, of growing up just to grow old, and to die. The turning point came when I accepted an invitation to attend a talk by an American evangelist who spoke about God and the Gospel. His message was simple but sincere. He sounded like he lived his talk. It dawned on me that I, like everyone else, needed God's grace and mercy. For the first time, I understood what the Gospel was about and I felt a keen sense of my unworthiness as I heard about God's compelling love. I also realised that I had no right to pass judgment on other Christians for their shortcomings. It was also during this time that I came to know Sue, an older person who befriended me and, through her ways and actions, personified God's love. I had on occasions seen her relating to people who needed her help. Her consistent care and concern for them without drawing attention to herself made an impact on me and helped restore my faith in Christians. Sue talked about her belief and faith with me in ways that I could understand.

One Sunday, after four years of missing church service, I returned to church. I decided to become a Christian and was baptised when I was 20 years old. It was a decision that I made for myself. I decided to believe in God because I wanted to, not because I had to.

I thought that I was doing well because I attended church and Bible studies. I even became a Sunday school teacher. As a result of my poor experience with my Sunday school teachers, I made sure that every child in my class received personal attention from me. I made it a point to chat with each student and get to know them better. I got married and went on to have three children. The issues I had to handle were relatively minor and easily managed. Because life was fairly stable, I was lulled into thinking that I was strong in my faith. I was living the Christian life and with God on my side, what challenges could I not manage and overcome?

Suicide, for one. I was thrown out of my comfort zone when Dad took his life. My Bible studies over the years did not prepare me for the hard questions that would hit me: Why did God allow this to happen to me? Why did He allow not just my Mum, but also my Dad, to take their lives? Was it a punishment? Was it a curse? Losing both my parents to suicide created a lot of questions regarding God's love and His claims of sovereignty. If His claims of omnipotence, omniscience and omnipresence were credible, why did He not stop my parents from taking their lives? Was He a loving God but powerless or a powerful God but lacking in loving kindness? I could quote Bible verses and spout "godly" platitudes when bad things happened to other people, but when Dad died, I was thrown into a crisis of faith. When Mum died through suicide, I had only two questions: Would she go to heaven? Would I see her again? I spoke to various people over the years about this issue and was satisfied with the answers I heard. However, when Dad died, also through suicide, I had to confront the issue of both my parents' suicides not only on the spiritual level, but also on an emotional level.

I ranted and raved at God. I struggled for months with conflicting thoughts and numerous questions. During this period, I was fortunate to have Tina with me, listening to my complaints and all the while loving me despite my being totally unlovable. Her acceptance and her non-judgmental ways were a reflection of God's love. We spent many hours talking about Dad's suicide, about the effects of the suicide on my family and me. We talked about God, my anger towards Him, and my inability to grasp God's way of working. Tina listened patiently, never speaking in defence of God. I guess she knew that God did not need defending. I appreciated the many hours she spent with me. She was comfortable with my silence, my anger, my tears. I also remember the numerous times Tina would provide me with tissues that were huge and durable, suitable for tears that flowed unceasingly.

Tina's supporting presence in my spiritual journey as a survivor was crucial for me to trust God again. It was not an overnight transformation that changed my mistrust to trust. rather, I had to make a conscious decision to trust God despite the situation that I was in. After struggling for sometime with the many unanswered questions, I finally accepted His will. I decided that my finite mind could never grasp the plan and purpose of an infinite God. In some inexplicable way, I started to feel less weary when I decided to "let go and let God".

One day, I was driving to some place. I thought of Dad and of his tragic death, and my eyes welled up. I missed him. Something caused me to look up at the sky and I started to sob. I saw some dark clouds with a silver lining. At that instant, I felt God saying something to me. up to that moment, since Dad's suicide, I had been focussing on myself and how miserable I was. That day, I was reminded that God was the creator of the universe, and that, as my creator, He knew the pain I was carrying. I was comforted by the thought, even though I could not logically explain the sense of peace I had experienced.

Some readers might find my journey of faith difficult to understand. It might even sound clichéd. But it was real for me; I had made a choice to believe that God was sovereign, and that His plans were for good though they might seem evil to me then.

Even now, I cannot understand God's purpose in allowing Dad and Mum's suicide to happen. For that reason, my journey will always be weighed down by doubts, a weak faith, and lots of tough questions. But I believe that, one day, all will be made known to me, when my journey on earth is over. In the meantime, there will be times when God will appear to be totally silent. There were numerous nights, following Dad's death, when I could not sleep well because of fear and anxiety. I remember crying out to God to give me sleep. Most nights, I would be a lot calmer and be able to drift off to sleep again, but there were nights when sleep eluded me. Sometimes, I experienced peace and His presence especially when I set aside time for quiet moments to reflect on God. Those were times when I would somehow reach a place when I reminded myself that God was still in charge-if silent-and that my decision to trust Him meant that I would keep walking with Him,

I was also able to find comfort in some Bible verses. A particularly helpful passage is 2nd Corinthians 12: 9. "My grace is sufficient for you, for my power is made perfect in weakness. " God does not promise that life will be free of challenges, but He says that in the midst of pain and confusion, He enables and He gives strength.

Other passages in the Bible were especially helpful in my journey too, such as the story of Job. Job was severely tested to a point where his faith in God was shaken to its very core. He lost his properties, his children, his health-everything! In no way was my hardship comparable to Job's, but his story showed me that affliction had a place in my life. Perhaps God had used Mum and Dad's suicide to speak to me. Perhaps it was His way of telling me to pause, take stock of my life, my relationships and my misplaced priorities. I was constantly running around, doing various urgent things at the expense of pursuing what was truly important. After Dad's death, I wished that I had spent more time with him. Certainly my relationship with him was more important than my myriads of urgent matters. Now, I try to spend more time nurturing relationships with my loved ones. Looking back, I am saddened that it had taken the loss of someone so precious to jolt me into not taking relationships for granted.

Time and again, God came through for me when I cried out to Him. If my life had been hunky dory, I would not be encountering God in such intimate ways. I might even forget God. I know that I will continue to struggle and to doubt God's goodness, but I also know, with some certainty, that God is much bigger than my doubts and fragile faith. He has promised that His grace is sufficient for me especially when I feel weak, helpless and hopeless.

Another positive that has resulted from my pain of loss is that I have become more empathetic and sensitive to other people and their loss. I used to be an extremely proud person, fiercely independent, refusing to rely on others. However, when I had to accept help from my counsellors and friends, I learnt humility. It also made me a better helper to other survivors, having been on the receiving end. I am now more balanced than before. Previously, my focus was on giving. Now, I have learnt to receive too. God was, and is using, the pain of Dad's suicide to help me be a better person.

Besides the Bible, other books also contributed to my personal growth during my crisis of faith. I was glad to have read Luci Shaw's God In The Dark. A friend had read it long ago and thought that I might find the book helpful. Luci Shaw, a speaker, poet, writer and editor, chronicled her husband's diagnosis and eventual death through cancer and of her own struggles as his caregiver. The author offers no pat answers, only an honest account of her difficulties in coming to terms with her pain and her grief. I found her honest questioning of God refreshing. Shaw's account of her doubt and anger with God showed me what a relationship with God should be like. Questioning God is not necessarily a lack of faith, but an exercise of faith.

C. S. Lewis, a philosopher and an author of science fiction, children's stories and Christian books, wrote in one of his books, The Problem Of Pain, that "God whispers to us in our pleasures, speaks to us in our conscience but shouts to us in our pain: it is His megaphone to rouse a deaf world. " I was very often hard of hearing or more accurately, selective in my hearing. I do not really know what brought it about. Perhaps it was more gratifying to be involved in activities that gave instant gratification. I pray and hope that God need not use His megaphone on me again, that I will be sensitive to His voice sans the megaphone.

Dan Allender, one of my favourite writers of Christian books, wrote in The Healing Path: "God confuses us as He allows harm and heart ache to enter our lives. But oddly, in the midst of loss, He also confirms His love in a way that is both mysterious and maddening. Maddening! God disturbs us and then woos us and wins us. " It sums up accurately what I want to say about my spiritual journey.

regardless of a survivor's background or faith, the struggles that he or she encounters are similar, even in the spiritual aspect. The sharing of my spiritual journey is by no means an indication that I have all the answers. I still struggle with questions regarding God's goodness and His purpose in allowing tragedies to happen. I know that as long as I am alive, I will be subjected to moods that will make me doubtful and even skeptical. My mood can and will vacillate according to external factors but I would like to think and believe that God is unchanging and constant.

While struggling towards healing, something was holding me back. It was my anger which kept coming up again and again during counselling sessions with Ophelia. We explored the reasons for my anger and talked about the need to forgive others and myself so that healing could begin. I agreed with her theoretically, but could find neither the strength nor the desire to do so. Although I wanted to release the anger, I was compelled to hold on to some of it. I felt entitled to be angry. I was adamant that I could not and did not want to force myself to forgive. I felt strongly that forgiveness must be motivated by a willingness and a desire to do so and that it could only happen when the wrongdoer was repentant. For me, the wrongdoers were all the people I was angry with. This issue was resolved one day when, after an especially difficult session with Ophelia, I went home very discouraged. All I had wanted to do on reaching home was to seek comfort in reading. It was and still is my way of entering another world temporarily to escape the reality of any difficult situations. A Longing For Home by Frederick Buechner caught my eye as I was longing for the home I had come to be associated with Dad. When Buechner was very young, his father had committed suicide. One of the chapters in the book titled The Journey Toward Wholeness conveyed the amazing grace of God extended to unworthy sinners. I began to understand the essence of forgiveness, something I had been trying to do for months. In his book, Buechner asked, "How is it possible in a broken world to become whole? Is wholeness something that we reach by taking pains, taking thoughts? Is it something that is given to us by grace alone? Is wholeness a human possibility at all?"

Buechner referred to the story of The Brothers Karamazov, as fictionalised by Dostoyevsky. "Zossima did not become a whole human being all in an instant as the novel goes to show. There is a long journey ahead of him still as there is a long journey ahead of all of us still. But the grace of God which reaches him through his vision of the beautiful day opens not just his eyes to see that life is heaven but opens his heart where heaven has dwelled all along. What Dostoyevsky tells us is that the journey towards wholeness for Zossima and for all of us is above all else a journey towards that capacity to love which is called compassion. "

Somehow, my anger was taken away that day. It was, and still is, a "miracle" for me to experience the transformation within my heart. My persistent anger, bitterness and resentment were, slowly but surely, replaced with a sense of love and sympathy towards those I was angry with. In place of anger, there was a tenderness of the heart. I did not have to force myself to forgive; instead, I was given a desire to do so. Perhaps, I saw how utterly unlovable I was and still am, and how much I myself needed forgiveness and grace, just like everyone else.

On the day of Dad's funeral, Tina gave me a letter. It was a source of comfort then and it makes even more sense now. This was what she wrote:

Dear Yin,

Two thoughts came to me this morning:

1 Your dad is no longer bound in that body of weakness and decay. He is now free from that, free to dance.

2 The people who loved Jesus must have felt the same as you do when He died. To them, it felt like the end. They could only see the darkness and despair, and feel the anguish that He had died such a tragic death.

But His death was not the end of the story. His death accomplished a purpose far greater than we can grasp. And the love that moved Him to suffer that death still holds us in thrall.

So even though we cannot see with eyes weary with tears and hearts and minds clouded by grief and pain, your dad and his story did not end with his dying. His life and the love you all bear for him (not just his children but also his children-in-law and grandchildren) are testimony to his life. He triumphed over such great adversity and brought up his children through the tragedy of your mother's death, through extreme financial hardship. He brought up a second generation of Christians and now there is a third.

It's impossible not to feel the terrible ache of your loss; because he was a loving father, the loss is so great. It'll take time. Maybe the ache will remain but it will not be the constant ache it now is.

God has not abandoned you. Your father has not abandoned you. His dying has caused so much pain. But I think, in his heart, he meant it for good.

I and all who love you are with you in this.

Tina

Chapter 6

How Time Heals

Old year, and then a new year,

It feels the same here, to me.

I ache, and I cry, And in many a sideway glance I try,

As if perchance, by slightest chance,

To catch a glimpse, however brief,

Of a figure that once was,

And still is, very dear to me.

Where can I go that he has not been?

My memory stalks me in every room I walk;

A painful longing

When my heart shapes a form

I cannot see, however hard I stare.

And yet I feel him peering from behind,

And I hear him climb the stairs.

He is everywhere in this house

But no longer here with me.

Living with memories

The moments slipped into days, weeks, months, and eventually into the first and second anniversaries of Dad's death. There is never a day that I do not think of my Dad. The memories remain with me — memories of how he was when he was alive; memories of his illness which caused him to feel helpless and distraught, and which often reduced him to tears of frustrations, fears and sadness; memories of the day he ended his life. I suspect they will remain with me for a long time to come. Time does bring healing, but it will never erase from my mind the father I loved and lost through suicide.

It amazes me that I can live without Dad's comforting presence in my life. Had I not reached out for support and affirmation from friends, fellow survivors, and SOS counsellors, I might still be reeling from the aftermath of his suicide. I am writing this book two years after he died, and I still miss him. But increasingly, I can recall and hold on to the happier memories I have of him. Occasionally, I feel his absence quite keenly and the pain of grief returns. Now and then, I cry. But it no longer overwhelms me. I remember his smile, his laughter, his voice. And I carry these memories of Dad in my heart and mind.

Like climbing a spiral staircase, I will continue to revisit feelings and issues, but from a different and hopefully higher plane each time. When he was alive and mobile, Dad used to spend a day at my place every week. In the immediate months after Dad's suicide, it was too unbearable to even think that he would never again spend time at my house. So I pushed those thoughts away whenever they came up. I did not want to remember his weekly presence in my house because his absence was too painful. Now, however, I recall these happy times and treasure the memories of him in my house. We did not do anything special but would usually spend the day doing ordinary things: watching his favourite TV programmes and cooking. He would make himself at home and just potter around the house and the garden and occasionally, he did a bit of gardening while I carried on with my household chores.

The same thing happened with my memories of our vacations overseas. About a year after Dad's suicide, I felt that I needed to take a vacation. I thought that if I went away for some time, I could leave the memories of Dad's suicide behind for a while, and take a break from the heaviness of grieving. But as it turned out, during the holiday, I had vivid memories of Dad and the time we spent on overseas trips, and I felt very sad because there would never be any more trips with him, ever again. The change in scenery was supposed to provide some respite from the constant reminders of my loss, and my husband and children worked hard to make it an enjoyable trip for me. Still, I kept recalling how it had been with Dad. I recalled helping him pack for the trip. He always travelled light but was careful to pack enough warm clothes because he was averse to the cold. I remembered how we had to take things slowly because Dad had, by then, become quite slow in his movements, yet doggedly refused any suggestion of using a wheelchair or even a walking cane. The economy seat on the plane was uncomfortable for his old bones, yet he never complained, and would eat whatever was served even though he had certain food preferences. On reaching the destination, he would rather stay indoors because of the cold, but with our encouragement, he would gallantly venture out. I would help him to bundle up so that he would not feel cold. And how meticulously he shopped for gifts for friends and family! These snippets of recollection during my vacation triggered intense sadness and a sense of loss again. It was not a good holiday for me.

But the second family vacation, a year later, felt different. We went to America where we had lived for a couple of years when my husband's work had taken him there. It sparked memories of when Dad had come for a visit. I thought of his response to the new place, the food, the cold weather and the people. But I was able to visualise Dad laughing, smiling and enjoying the moments of family togetherness. Most of all, I remember the look of contentment and pride on his face as he spoke about his family with friends and relatives overseas.

Milestones

Although it is a struggle for survivors to move on, I found that we do encounter certain milestones in our journey of grief. I went for counselling in the hope that it might somehow hasten my journey and, hopefully, be healed by the first anniversary of my dad's suicide; that if I could get through the first year I would be all right; that my life would go back to normal. That was the milestone that I had set for myself. Of course it turned out to be a false marker. I now know, from my own experience and from hearing other survivors, that the milestones are not dictated by time. Some survivors pass certain milestones sooner than others and the milestones might differ for each survivor. But there were some milestones that my fellow survivors and I had in common.

Ending intrusive recalls

One of my milestones was the disappearance of intrusive recalls. During the initial period of grief, I kept thinking of the last day I saw my dad alive. I kept seeing him in my mind, how I had helped him sit up in bed that morning because he no longer had the strength to sit up by himself. And how he said "OK" as I was leaving. That image and the resonance of that "OK" kept replaying in my head. I had no control over when it would replay. Then one day, these intrusive recalls just stopped. I cannot remember when it happened but I do know that, these days, I have to recall the scene intentionally when I want to revisit those memories: they no longer pop into my head. I do revisit them sometimes because I do not want to lose the memory of my last day with my Dad. Now and then, I summon up the memories as a way to tenderise my heart a reminder to be empathetic towards other survivors who were just starting on their journey.

I also noticed that the memory of that last day was no longer as painful as it used to be. In the beginning, the recall was accompanied by a lot of negative feelings, especially regret and guilt. But these negative feelings have become less cutting now and guilt has almost disappeared. Two years after the suicide, I can comfortably say that I had done what I could to the best of my ability at that time.

I can now also recall and stay longer with the good memories—our outings together, the trips we made overseas, watching TV in his company, and his presence in my car whenever I took him out. In the first few months after the suicide, whenever I tried to recall the good memories of my dad, it would send me into a tailspin of "if only" and back to the bad memories.

In the beginning, I needed to visit Dad's niche every week as a way of maintaining some connection with him. After the first anniversary I was able to space out my visits; I went mainly on special occasions. I did not have to be there to maintain a connection with Dad. When I need to remember him, I just look in my heart and mind.

Tony, another survivor who had lost his father to suicide, had had a similar experience with memories. In the initial months after his father jumped, he had constant replays of their last conversation and of the moment when he received word of the tragedy. He found that after several sessions with the counsellor, he was able to stop the intrusive thoughts of his father's suicide. And when those thoughts stopped intruding, he could think and manage the other aspects of his grief better. He also stopped making daily trips to the niche to be with his father.

Fewer triggers

Mrs. Wong spoke of how, in the past, she had taken pains to avoid people who might trigger memories of her son. She avoided her nephews and her friends who had children of the same age. But three years later, she could be in the same room as they and even say hello, though she still could not hold a conversation with them.

I had a similar experience with people and places that were triggers for me. Initially, I could not bear to meet my siblings; I was afraid that just seeing them would bring back the painful memories of how we were at the apartment after the suicide, at the wake and at the funeral. About a year and a half later, I no longer felt so dreadful when I had to meet my siblings for family occasions. We still did not talk about Dad's suicide, but I no longer needed to avoid them.

Sometimes, certain things cease to be triggers. These days I can walk past Dad's barbershop without feeling pained by memories of his suicide. I may momentarily think of him, but the thought passes quickly and I can continue doing whatever has taken me there in the first place. I have also gone back to my usual fishmonger because he is no longer a trigger, though these days I naturally buy less fish without Dad around.

Reaching out

Some of us have reached a point in our journey when we can help others without being overwhelmed by our own pain. The tragedy has made us more sensitive to other people in distress and there is a deep desire to help. Mrs Wong reported how, in the course of her work, she could connect with a total stranger who had lost his mother to illness. He found her responses so heartwarming, and he commended her to her boss. Sheila stopped to listen to and comfort a neighbour whose mother died from illness. She wondered whether she would have made the extra effort if she had not experienced her own painful loss. Lian and Joanne willingly became co-facilitators at the Healing Bridge and they also made themselves available to survivors during their personal time outside of the Healing Bridge sessions. They still cry during the sharing sessions, but they have become strong enough to comfort new survivors.

About one-and-a-half years into my journey of grief, Ophelia asked me to co-facilitate the Healing Bridge sessions with her. I readily agreed, as I believed in the affirming work of the group sessions. That was an important milestone for me, because I was finally ready to walk with other survivors and carry my own pain as well.

In 2007, for the first time in my life, I spoke publicly about my tragedy. SOS had organised a forum for survivors of suicide so that they could hear the experiences of veteran survivors. I agreed to be part of a panel of four Healing Bridge members to share our stories and answer questions about how we coped. We also wanted the new survivors to know that they were not alone in their grief, that they could find support here. Knowing that I was not alone was a critical factor in my healing, I was prepared to be somewhat less mindful of my privacy if it could help other survivors. The tragedy of suicide happens to other people too—people who are good parents and children, whose loved ones committed suicide. I cried as I shared my story with the nearly two dozen new survivors present. At the same time, I was also glad that I could play a part in helping them understand what they were going through and inviting them to join the support group.

Not the end

My experience as a suicide survivor is like setting out on a journey against my will. At the start of the journey, I hoped to arrive at a destination where all would be well, where the past would be left behind and the journey would be over and I could once again look forward to the future which I envisaged to be bright and happy again. I have since learnt that my journey is ongoing; it's a life-long journey.

Helen Keller, a remarkable American woman, was born blind and deaf, but against all odds, she learnt to speak, read and write. She said: "What we have once enjoyed we can never lose. All that we have loved deeply becomes a part of us. " I first saw these words on a brochure from the SOS. I was comforted by the thought that although Dad was no longer around, his values and all he stood for, live on in my memories and in my life.

In that sense—in a very real sense—Dad will always live in and through me.

Acknowledgments

To my husband and children, for the times when I was physically present but emotionally absent, I want to express my thanks for your love, understanding and encouragement.

To Tina my dear friend, for walking with me right from the very beginning of my journey and even now, thank you. Without your friendship, patience and love, this journey might have taken me to a very different place.

To Ophelia Ooi my counsellor from SOS, your perseverance and patience never fail to amaze me. Thank you for believing in me, guiding me and giving me the confidence to complete the book and in the process helping me to believe that good can emerge from the pain of losing my parents to suicide.

To my fellow survivors, thank you for being my fellow sojourners in this journey. Your courage to live on and your desire to help other survivors inspire me.

To God, even though I cannot yet see your purpose in allowing these tragic events to happen, I am grateful for the moments when I experienced your peace in the midst of excruciating pain and turmoil.

About the author

When she was only 7, yin's mother took her own life. Forty years later her father jumped to his death. This is the story of how she survived her parents' suicides. Yin, 47 was a physiotherapist before becoming a homemaker. She is married with 3 children, aged 20, 18 and 16.